Managing Stress and Preventing Burnout in the Healthcare Workplace

Managing Stress

and Preventing

Burnout in the

Healthcare Workplace

Jonathon R. B. Halbesleben

HAP

ACHE Management Series

Your board, staff, or clients may also benefit from this book's insight. For more information on quantity discounts, contact the Health Administration Press Marketing Manager at (312) 424-9470.

This publication is intended to provide accurate and authoritative information in regard to the subject matter covered. It is sold, or otherwise provided, with the understanding that the publisher is not engaged in rendering professional services. If professional advice or other expert assistance is required, the services of a competent professional should be sought.

The statements and opinions contained in this book are strictly those of the author(s) and do not represent the official positions of the American College of Healthcare Executives or of the Foundation of the American College of Healthcare Executives.

14   13   12   11   10   5   4   3   2   1

Library of Congress Cataloging-in-Publication Data

Halbesleben, Jonathon R. B.
  Managing stress and preventing burnout in the healthcare workplace /
Jonathon R. B. Halbesleben.
     p. cm.
  Includes bibliographical references and index.
  ISBN 978-1-56793-343-7 (alk. paper)
  1. Medical personnel--Mental health. 2. Stress management. 3. Burn
out (Psychology) I. Title.

  RC451.4.M44H35 2009
  362.196'98--dc22

                          2009038621

The paper used in this publication meets the minimum requirements of American National Standard for Information Sciences—Permanence of Paper for Printed Library Materials, ANSI Z39.48-1984. ∞™

Found an error or a typo? We want to know! Please e-mail it to hap1@ache.org, and put "Book Error" in the subject line.

For photocopying and copyright information, please contact Copyright Clearance Center at www.copyright.com or (978) 750-8400.

Project manager: Jennifer Seibert; Acquisitions editor: Janet Davis; Cover designer: Scott Miller

Health Administration Press
A division of the Foundation
   of the American College of
   Healthcare Executives
One North Franklin Street
Suite 1700
Chicago, IL 60606
(312) 424-2800

For Jenn, Alex, and Liesl—my unconditional sources of social support

Contents

Acknowledgments ix

Introduction: The Role of the Healthcare Manager in Addressing
    Stress and Burnout xi

Chapter 1: Making the Case for Addressing Stress and Burnout in
    Healthcare Organizations 1

Chapter 2: Defining the Problem of Stress and Burnout in
    Healthcare Organizations 17

Chapter 3: When Stress Becomes Burnout 33

Chapter 4: Capturing Stress and Burnout 43

Chapter 5: The BRIDGES Program: Reducing Burnout in
    Healthcare Professionals 53

Chapter 6: Taking Sustainability to the Next Level: Developing a
    "Stress-Free Environment" 79

Chapter 7: Putting It All Together: Beating Burnout, Building
    Engagement 95

Appendix A: Helpful Resources for Dealing with
    Stress and Burnout 101

Appendix B: BRIDGES Resources 107

References 111

Index 117

About the Author 123

Acknowledgments

PROJECTS SUCH AS this one may end up single-authored, but require a significant unseen group effort to produce. I have many people to thank for assisting me in this endeavor.

My family, particularly my wonderful wife, Jenn, and our children, has had an extraordinarily supportive role in my ability to write this book. I made the potentially unwise decision, with the benefit of hindsight, to write a book while my wife and I were expecting a child. Our daughter arrived shortly before my deadline. As such, many of the chapters were written while holding a small baby in the early morning hours. My wife has always been amazing in her support of my career endeavors, no matter how ambitious or minor, and for that I will always be grateful. Also, special thanks to Carol Gordon and Leslie Lyons—their help allowed me to finish this project.

My research collaborators over the years have inspired many of the ideas presented in this book. I particularly thank Tony Wheeler (University of Rhode Island), Matt Bowler (Oklahoma State University), Mike Buckley (University of Oklahoma), Doug Wakefield (University of Missouri), Bonnie Wakefield (Iowa City VA Medical Center), Cheryl Rathert (University of Missouri) and Mike Mumford (University of Oklahoma).

Tim Vaughan, chair of the Department of Management and Marketing, and Tom Dock, dean of the College of Business, of the University of Wisconsin–Eau Claire have provided me a great deal of instrumental support that has allowed me to complete this project. The staff of the UW–Eau Claire Office of Sponsored Programs and Research, in particular Karen Havholm and Roger Wareham, has been critical in facilitating the financial support for my research. Their support has permitted me to explore stress and burnout with the depth needed to offer meaningful advances in the literature.

Janet Davis, Jennifer Seibert, and the staff at Health Administration Press have made this a far better book than I could have ever produced alone. Their tireless behind-the-scenes work to produce such high-quality work is admirable.

Thanks to Ryan and Laura of the Goat Coffeehouse and the folks at the Coffee Grounds in Eau Claire, Wisconsin, for giving me a refuge in which to write much of this book. It has inspired me to study the stress-relieving effects of good coffee and good company, if only through self-reflection.

I wish to thank the healthcare professionals who informed this book. My work, whether through interviews, observations, or surveys, has put me in contact with literally thousands of healthcare professionals over the last few years. I thank them for their candor in sharing their experiences with me. While the milieu with regard to stress has shifted toward accepting that stress is inevitable in healthcare, it still requires a great deal of courage to share and relive the stress in one's life.

Finally, while it is incredibly cliché, I want to thank you, the reader. If you are reading this book, you recognize that stress and burnout are having an impact on those you work with. More important, it suggests you have the audacity to do something about it! Clearly, you have some hope that you can address the stress problems in your facility. My hope is that, by the end of this book, I have energized that hope so you can tackle the problem, which I will argue is an epidemic, head-on. It will be a challenging journey. Thank you for the opportunity to lead you in that journey.

The Role of the Healthcare Manager in Addressing Stress and Burnout

Welcome to the most stressful floor in the hospital.
    —Nurse working in a cardiac intensive care unit
      in a major academic medical center

I'm so glad you are conducting your research here. This is the most stressful place to work in the hospital!
    —Nurse working in the pediatric intensive care unit
      of the same academic medical center

I'M MORE STRESSED THAN YOU ARE!

I have an odd hobby (or, if you like, call it an obsession). I like lists—a lot. This book started as a list of stuff I planned to write about. I added items from that list to my to-do list. My to-do list often includes things I know I will do without having to remind myself, but I include them solely because I enjoy checking things off the list! Today I read an online story about the top ten worst contracts in baseball history. On television tonight, my wife and I will probably be drawn into some list about celebrities or home improvement. I also compile lists about the lists I like.

Among my favorites are the lists of stressful jobs. While their methodology is often dubious, popular publications now commonly release lists of the most stressful jobs. Healthcare administrators and others interested in the field will not be surprised that healthcare jobs frequently reside near the top of the lists. *Health* magazine recently included medical internships in its top ten. A list of the United Kingdom's top ten most stressful jobs included ambulance service (#5), nursing (#6), medicine (#7), and dentistry (#9). Other lists include surgery and nursing home jobs. A consistent theme emerges from these lists: People working in healthcare seem to be pretty stressed out. But lists are only part of the story.

Perhaps more interesting about these lists are the comments they elicit. Such lists draw strong emotional reactions, likely because the jobs of those in healthcare are so core to their personal identity. For example, on one website that posted *Health* magazine's list, readers left a litany of comments: *How could firefighting not be at the top of the list? What about anesthesiology? An anesthesiologist's decision could cost someone his life! Teaching is listed, but only for inner-city high schools; what about the rest of us?*

These comments are interesting, not so much because of the occupations that might be missed or over-/underrated, but because they highlight a familiar theme: We all find our jobs stressful at times. Moreover, we may have a hard time putting the stress or our job into perspective. I can give a personal example: One of the lists included natural and social scientist, but as one of the *least* stressful jobs. My immediate reaction was the same as that expressed by those who left comments about *Health* magazine's list: *Are you kidding me? How could you not have included it near the top? I'm dealing with student demands, managing grants, preparing for teaching, and research (and book!) deadlines, among other things.*

This response is natural. Imagine if you trained for years to learn how to do your job and had been working in the job for even longer. Then, someone tells you your job isn't stressful. Rationally, we should probably say, "Thank you—it's not stressful because I'm competent and able to manage my stress well." You likely wouldn't react that way, however. Stress has become something of a badge of honor in today's society. We expect our jobs to be stressful because that means we are working hard. It means our job is important, and that we have responsibilities. It means we are not replaceable cogs in a machine but critical points in a system. As a result, when someone hints that our job isn't stressful, we lash out. We argue our point. We post our rebuttal for all of cyberspace to read. With the advent of the Internet, communication has become easier. As noted earlier, most news stories include an area where comments can be posted. There is a Yahoo! group dedicated to discussing the most stressful jobs. Forums have been set up on other sites for this purpose (e.g., on nurse.com). Finally, there are numerous Facebook groups dedicated to professing the stressful nature of jobs.

In their book about stress among physicians in England, David Wainwright and Michael Calnan (2002) argued that there has been an interesting shift in how people react to stress over the past century. Whereas jobs were arguably more labor intensive and less safe years ago, people seem more likely to report stress now than ever before. Evidence from the academic study of stress supports their argument. Stress was not even a topic of study in areas such as psychology until the 1940s. Before that point, it was strictly an engineering term, and people rarely talked about how stressed they were. *Stress* was a term reserved for the effect of forces on bridges and other structures.

Are we really more stressed than people were 50 years ago? It seems unlikely. Our attitudes toward work and our reactions to it have changed, however. Self-identifying as a stressed-out martyr is much more popular than it once was.

Whether stress is a "real" effect or just an artifact of how we like to identify with our work, we would be silly to dismiss the stress epidemic as a passing fad. Even if we would prefer to take that approach, too much evidence suggests we had better not ignore it. We are quickly realizing that people who experience stress (and who report experiencing stress) act in ways that can be problematic for their organizations and for their own well-being. Over the long term, what starts as a relatively minor complaint can blossom into burnout, lower performance, and even turnover and violence.

In this sense, this text is not a self-help book. Let's face it—if we could help ourselves, stress wouldn't be considered an epidemic. Rather, this text is an "other-help" book. **The goal of this book is to put you, as a practicing healthcare administrator, in a better position to address the stress of those with whom you work.** Altruistically, you will seem like a caring manager when you exercise the knowledge you have gained. Professionally, this insight could benefit your organization dramatically in terms of smoother functioning and better bottom-line performance. Selfishly, you will look like a much better administrator! Let's start by defining this ubiquitous concept of stress in terms of what it is and what it is not.

WHAT STRESS IS

Stress is more difficult to define than one might imagine. It is one of those ideas that people can identify when they see it but would be hard-pressed to pinpoint in words. Researchers have debated the definition of stress for many years, and a consensus has yet to emerge.

What makes stress so hard to define is a lack of clarity about whether we are talking about a state of being, an event, a process, or something else altogether. For example, when people say they are "stressed," do they mean they are experiencing a state of stressfulness? Or do they mean they have just experienced an acute event that they interpreted as negative? Or do they mean they are using some sort of cognitive process to compare their current situation to their desired situation (and are presumably reaching an unfavorable conclusion)?

The National Institute for Occupational Safety and Health (NIOSH) has been a leading government agency in the study of stress in the United States. In its seminal report, *Stress at Work,* NIOSH (1999) defines job stress as "the harmful physical and emotional responses that occur when the requirements of the job do not match the capabilities, resources, or needs of the worker."

In a way, NIOSH's definition summarizes the three possibilities noted in the previous paragraph. By including the idea of a response to a stimulus, the definition highlights the cognitive process as well as the acute event (consideration of the requirements of the job).

A critical aspect of NIOSH's definition is the cognitive evaluation that underlies stress. This evaluation has long been a focus of stress theorists, who believe that just tallying up someone's stressful experiences (which we will refer to as *stressors*) does not help us understand how stress is experienced. As a result of this conviction, the life event scales that were popularized early on as a way to determine stress—on which you checked off whether you received a promotion, got divorced, got married, had a child, and had a major death in the family—have fallen out of favor. We now recognize that our reactions to these events, rather than the events themselves, are potentially more problematic.

In summary, stress is a state of being that results from our evaluation of a specific situation. It is our response when we face a demand at work but do not feel we have sufficient resources to meet the demand.

WHAT STRESS IS NOT

In addition to defining what stress is, it may also be helpful to clarify what stress is not. A number of constructs are similar to stress, and indeed related to stress, but should not be confused for stress. Dissatisfaction, lack of commitment, and incompetence are three such concepts.

Stress Is Not Dissatisfaction

Stress is not the same as dissatisfaction with work. Someone highly satisfied with his work could be stressed because he spends so much time worrying about aspects of his job. Positive, satisfying events at work (e.g., promotions) can also be stressful.

Over time, stress can lead to dissatisfaction. As stress mounts, people will eventually react negatively to it. People expect some level of stress in their jobs, but when it seems inescapable, they reach a point where they become dissatisfied with the job.

Stress Is Not Lack of Commitment

The same thinking applies to one's commitment to work. Extreme commitment to work might be causing the stress. An employee who repeatedly experiences stress will slowly detach from her job. In essence, she will begin to question whether her values truly align with the organization's values.

Stress Is Not Incompetence

People who experience stress aren't incompetent. If not carefully considered, the NIOSH definition might lead one to that conclusion (e.g., the requirements of the job don't meet the capabilities of the worker). However, one also needs to consider the rest of the definition—the needs of the worker and the resources available to the worker. The person might be highly capable of doing his job but does not find that it meets his needs. He may not be earning enough from the job and thus cannot meet his material needs. Or, it might not be providing the psychosocial stimulation he seeks. Under these circumstances, a competent person may still experience a great deal of stress.

The definition also cites insufficient resources to meet the requirements of the job. I'll define *resources* more carefully later in the book, but for now, I'll just say that resources can include nearly anything—time, financial support, assistance from colleagues, equipment—the list goes on. This problem is readily apparent to many nurses: They would like to spend more time with each of their patients, but staffing crunches have increased the number of patients assigned to them. As result, they feel as though they are not meeting the requirements of the job, at least to the extent they would like to meet them. Again, the issue is not one of incompetence; they just do not have the resources they need to meet the demands of the job.

THE STRESS PARADOX

One of the difficulties in addressing stress is something I will refer to as the *stress paradox*: for the most part, stress processes are personal, subjective experiences. However, when we want to reduce stress, individual interventions are not particularly effective. Why? The answer to that question is key to this book. If we can understand why individuals uniquely experience stress (for example, why one colleague thrives on short deadlines while another finds them debilitating) and why individual interventions don't work, we will move much closer to addressing the problem of stress in the workplace. In this section, I outline the basic arguments for the stress paradox as a way to present the assumptions on which this book is built.

Everyone Experiences Stress, but Not Everyone Experiences Burnout

We know that stress is an individual experience. As a result, while we all experience stress, we do not all experience the intense strain that characterizes burnout. *Burnout* is an extreme response to work stress that occurs when we continually face stressors with which we are unable to fully cope. Most people will react to stressors by concluding (at least initially) that they don't have adequate resources to meet the demand. However, the percentage of people who would be characterized as burned out is much lower. Some of us are able to deal with the stressors in life and stop them from becoming so bad that they burn us out. If some people can mitigate stress themselves, don't we have all the more reason to treat stress individually? On the surface, this logic seems sound, but let's dig a little deeper.

The Commonality of Stressors

While the experience of stress varies from person to person, we find remarkable consistency among the variation. When surveys are conducted in departments or common work areas (e.g., a floor in a hospital), the stressors that people name are often the same. The levels of burnout also tend to be highly consistent. Thus, while people may react somewhat differently to the stressors, employees working together typically react negatively to the same stressors. For example, when staffing is a problem, it is a problem for everyone. These data explain why treating this problem individually won't work. Imagine telling a nurse in an intensive care unit (ICU) that the staffing issue is not really that big of a deal and that he should think about it as an opportunity to show his value, or that staffing wouldn't be an issue if he managed his time better. Simply telling someone to reframe his problem won't make it go away, especially if everyone else is observing the same problem. As hard as that nurse might try to think about short staffing as an opportunity, he is still going to struggle to get the work done and is still going to hear about the problem repeatedly.

People Know What Is Causing Their Stress, and They Likely Know the Solution, Too

The final assumption of this book, and arguably the key to addressing stress at work, is that employees know what is causing it. If you approach the subject delicately with them, you'll be able to solicit this information, and if you are smart, you'll ask them how they would fix the situation. Countless well-intentioned stress management programs have failed because managers thought they knew what was causing stress in the workplace and came up with a flashy seminar to address it. These managers may have wanted to show off their expertise and leadership ability, or perhaps they didn't want to bother their employees by soliciting their feedback. More likely, they did so because they (1) feared what they might discover and (2) feared that their employees would come up with solutions that they, as the manager, could not implement. A goal of this book is to convince you that such thinking is extremely problematic and is actually contributing further to the problem of stress in healthcare.

YOUR ROLE IN ADDRESSING STRESS

The final assumption places some of the responsibility for addressing stress on your employees. In other words, they should come up with the real solutions, right? Such thinking may initially make your role in the process muddy. Understand, however, that while employees have the solutions, they often wait for someone to ask them about them. They will need your help in developing detailed action plans for implementing the solutions. You will help build the framework that allows for long-term sharing of ideas and implementation of those ideas.

PLAN FOR THE BOOK

With your role in mind, this book will lead you down a path that should put you in a better position to address the stress you and your employees face regularly. To that end, we'll start by making the business case for addressing stress. I will convince you that not dealing with stress is far more costly than addressing it head-on. Then, we'll examine why people in healthcare experience such high stress and burnout and identify the source of that stress. We'll focus on burnout because it represents the point at which the stress becomes debilitating. From there, we will discuss strategies for reducing the burnout that employees are experiencing and for preventing future burnout. By the conclusion of the book, you will be more able to help your employees reverse the burnout they are experiencing and reengage them in their work.

CHAPTER 1

Making the Case for Addressing Stress and Burnout in Healthcare Organizations

I realized on day one that my job was going to be more stressful than I had anticipated. For a while I tried to deal with it, to cope, I guess. But after a few months, I just couldn't take it anymore.
—Former physical therapist working in a community hospital, now working as an insurance claims representative

School really sucks right now; it is totally stressful. But it will all get better once I get through med school and the residency program, right?
—Third-year medical student

WHY YOU NEED TO CARE ABOUT STRESS AND BURNOUT AMONG YOUR STAFF

Stress is an easy thing to ignore. It seems normal. Everyone is stressed, right? If you aren't a little stressed, are you really doing your job? In some ways, the answer to both of these questions is *yes*. Even the earliest stress theorists and researchers concluded that some level of stress (or perhaps better framed as "arousal") was required to accomplish daily activities. When I teach my students about stress, I will often tell them that their mere state of wakefulness means that they are experiencing stress.

However, we also know that too much stress can cause problems. In this chapter, I will review the significant impact that stress can have on healthcare professionals and administrative staff. Essentially, I will make a business case for caring about stress among healthcare staff. My goal isn't to tug at your heartstrings by arguing that a caring manager needs to worry about how stressed his staff is. That might be true, but there is also a link between stress and your purse strings. For better or worse, today's healthcare managers are more likely to pay attention to the financial argument. I am convinced that after I lay out these consequences, you will also be convinced that stress and, in its extreme form, burnout are issues that you need to strongly consider because of the impact on *both* your heartstrings and your purse strings.

COMMON CONSEQUENCES OF STRESS AMONG HEALTHCARE PROFESSIONALS

I hesitate to lump clinical and administrative professionals together when sorting out the negative impact of stress. As outlined in the Introduction, not everyone experiences stress in the same way. Moreover, as discussed in the next chapter, the sources of stress vary according to the type of clinical work. However, when we study the impact of stress on the working professional, we see that the patterns are remarkably consistent.

Burnout Leads to Lower Performance

One of the more consistent findings in the literature is that stress, especially when it reaches the point of burnout, has a negative impact on job performance. Performance is considered a multiplicative function of one's ability and motivation. In other words, to perform a job, one has to have the ability (e.g., the requisite skills and knowledge) and motivation to do the job. Research has established that decrements in performance are the result of decreased motivation. When employees are burned out, they retain the ability to do the work, but their desire to complete the work markedly declines. Consider the implications of this finding for a moment: We have a workforce that has the ability to do the job, but has little desire to do so. What a waste of human potential!

The underlying reason for the lack of motivation is essentially a resource allocation problem. In the introductory chapter, I introduced the idea that stress results from a mismatch between the demands of the job and the resources available to meet those demands. When we face demands at work, we allocate some of our resources to meet each new demand we face. When a new patient is transferred to a floor, the nurses on that floor have a new set of demands that will utilize their time, skills, material resources, even physical energy (in terms of burned calories). We repeatedly make decisions about how we will allocate or invest our resources.

What we tend to find is that people allocate their resources strategically. As their resources are diminished, they invest more carefully and in ways that are more likely to pay off in the long term. For example, when we aren't burned out, we may not think twice about helping another employee who seems to be having trouble. We may take a little more time to double-check our work (e.g., check a medication order twice to make sure the dosage is correct). But as our stress increases to the point where our resources are severely diminished, we have to allocate our resources more carefully. Suddenly, we're not sure whether we have the time to help that colleague, or we assume everything is okay with that medication order.

Burnout Affects How Work Gets Done

This resource allocation process has important implications for how work gets done in healthcare organizations. Recently, I've been spending a lot of time conducting research on the concept of workarounds—creative solutions for addressing blocks in workflow. I am finding that healthcare professionals are constantly dealing with blocks in their work. Equipment cannot be found where they thought it should be, patients' charts are missing information, or medication orders were not filled properly. Some of these blocks may be intentional, such as the forcing functions embedded in bar code medication administration technologies that make the employee stop and think about what he is doing.

However, when an employee is burned out, these blocks are interpreted differently. For example, scanning the medication and armband in a bar code medication administration system is not a big deal when stress is low. But in the face of burnout, a nurse might feel that the task is inconvenient and taking up her valuable time. Some nurses make copies of the patient armbands and place them close to the medications to eliminate repeated trips to the bedside for scanning. This shortcut saves them a little time as they administer medications, but it also eliminates the safety advantage that was built into the bar code system.

We have applied this idea not only to patient safety, but also to the safety of the healthcare professional. In the same way that nurses (and other professionals) may work around patient safety features, they may shortcut safety procedures meant to protect themselves. Our research is finding that when nurses experience higher levels of burnout, they engage in risky practices, such as not asking for assistance when moving patients. As a result, they increase their possibility of incurring occupational injuries, such as musculoskeletal damage.

Taken together, I am suggesting that when stress mounts, healthcare professionals strategically reallocate their resources in ways that allow them to do their job more efficiently (from their perspective) but that may also sub-optimize their outcomes. If they are reallocating their resources repeatedly, they may come to feel that they are not a good fit for the job.

Burnout Leads to Higher Turnover Intentions

Turnover intentions are the next potential consequence. Burnout is strongly linked to negative consequences such as job dissatisfaction, lower commitment, and eventual turnover. High levels of stress are shocks to an employee's system. Most healthcare professionals have spent a significant amount of time training for their professions. While that training might have been stressful, it is typically completed with the idea that it will pay off in the end when they land that first "real" job. When they take that job and realize that their stress might be much worse than anticipated, they begin to think about alternatives. Professionals may wonder whether they took the wrong job, or whether they took the wrong career path altogether. As a result, they start thinking about other options and may even begin a job search.

This effect appears to be particularly pronounced among early career (especially first-year) professionals, among whom research consistently finds higher levels of burnout and a stronger burnout–turnover relationship. If someone is really burned out, he or she is unlikely to stick around for a long time. In many of the healthcare professions, this factor has contributed to the well-documented staffing shortages. The perfect storm of baby boomers' retirement, high early-career turnover, and inadequate space in training programs presents an imminent crisis in most healthcare professions. While this issue is beyond the scope of this book, addressing stress may at least improve the retention part of the equation.

Burnout Is Harmful to Health

A growing body of literature supports the idea that job stress is negatively associated with health. For example, a study of 21,000 female nurses by researchers at Harvard University found that job-related strain is as harmful to health as smoking or a sedentary lifestyle (Cheng et al. 2000). We all recognize the dangers of smoking in the workplace, to the point where most healthcare organizations disallow it on campus. We regularly hear about smoke-free workplaces, so why don't we hear more about stress-free workplaces?

A leading researcher on this topic, Arie Shirom, has consistently found relationships between burnout and poor health. For example, in a 2006 review of the literature, Melamed, Shirom, and colleagues reported that burnout was as great a risk factor for cardiovascular disease as more traditional risk factors like smoking, high body mass index, and high blood pressure. Their work (as well as the work of others) has established a variety of physiological processes linking stress with cardiovascular disease.

Burnout has been associated with other negative health outcomes as well, including lower-rated self-health, type 2 diabetes, male infertility, and sleep disturbances. As this research becomes more popular and more sophisticated, the findings are revealing that burnout has a greater impact on occupational health than initially realized. Of course, this research is also focused on the mechanisms underlying the health concerns, but the bottom line is that high levels of stress have a negative impact on our bodies.

Individual Consequences of Stress and Burnout

- Decreased performance
- Potentially problematic (and even dangerous) adjustments to work process
- Higher turnover intention
- Poor health

One way of explaining some of these negative health outcomes is to look at how stress affects what we eat. A 2007 survey sponsored by the American Psychological Association found that eating "too much or bad foods" was a common coping mechanism of those facing stress. As you might imagine, people aren't binging on celery sticks and apples. Nearly two-thirds of the respondents indicated that candy or chocolate was their coping food of choice, followed closely by ice cream, potato chips, cookies, and cake (American Psychological Association 2007, 10). In view of these data, the link between stress and symptoms of diabetes and cardiovascular disease is not surprising.

Vicious Cycles

As if the above consequences weren't enough, emerging research suggests that those who are burned out tend to enter a vicious cycle that makes their burnout worse over time. The idea is pretty straightforward: As our resources are depleted, we are left with fewer options for investing our remaining resources; thus, we are more likely to lose those resources. For example, if we have barely enough resources to do our job, we are not likely to exhibit extra behaviors that would make us a more likely candidate for promotion. As a result, we are stuck in a job that is draining our resources.

Through research funded by the National Institute for Occupational Safety and Health, I am exploring this effect in regard to burnout, workarounds, and occupational safety. While the results are preliminary, they suggest that burned-out nurses are more likely to engage in workarounds. As a result, they are more likely to be injured on the job, which leads them to be even more burned-out and more likely to engage in workarounds. You can see how this downward cycle could lead to significant long-term problems.

The good news is that we can use these cycles to our advantage at times. We can also create virtuous cycles with resources if we can attain a critical mass of resources. Employees then can allocate their resources in a way that continually generates new resources. When this model is achieved, the result is a highly engaged workforce. We will return this idea later, as it will be critical in tackling the epidemic of stress in healthcare.

THE IMPACT ON ORGANIZATIONAL PERFORMANCE

The impact that stress has on organizational performance is the least clear part of the equation. While stress certainly has a marked effect on healthcare professionals as described above, research that sorts out the relationships between stress and its effects is difficult to conduct for many reasons. One reason is that stress has a delayed effect on organizations. Stress may build among employees for years until the full cost of stress is realized. Such reasons make causal research designs at the organizational level nearly impossible to implement. However, if we extend our discussion of the impact of stress to individuals, the organizational-level consequences quickly become clear.

We have already made the connection between burnout and outcomes, such as the link between performance and turnover discussed earlier. These outcomes have real costs in terms of human resource losses. The lost productivity associated with lower performance is pronounced. While no figures specific to healthcare are available, the American Institute of Stress (2009) estimates the cost of stress to be more than $300 billion in the U.S. economy alone. This figure is largely based on accidents, absenteeism, reduced productivity, medical costs, worker's compensation claims, and other costs directly associated with stress. Again, while this figure is for the entire United States, if we use a conservative estimate of 15 percent to represent the portion of the U.S. economy represented by healthcare, we still would be talking about $20 billion. Imagine how that money could be used constructively in the healthcare sector.

Turnover

A good bit of that $20 billion comes from costs associated with turnover. When someone quits his job, there are costs associated with recruiting and selecting someone to fill the position, training that new person once he takes the job, and lost productivity while the former employee is off the job (including lost clinical income in some cases) and the new employee is tackling the learning curve. These associated costs don't even include the more indirect costs associated with lower morale when someone vacates a position.

Of course, the costs associated with turnover vary significantly depending on the occupation. To summarize the impact, selected average replacement costs for a variety of healthcare professions are included in Exhibit 1.1. While the figures vary on the basis of a significant number of factors (e.g., local economy, supply and demand in the profession), they provide a useful illustration of the costs associated with turnover.

The numbers also should be put in a proper perspective based on turnover rates. For example, one study from the University of Arizona found that its medical and surgical departments had an *average* annual cost associated with turnover that exceeded $400,000 for a four-year period (fiscal years 2000–2004). The study found individual replacement costs to be as high as $587,125 for a surgical sub-

---

Exhibit 1.1 Costs Associated with Replacing Selected Employees (by Occupation/Specialty)

Physician
Generalist[1]	$115,554
Subspecialist[1]	$286,503
Surgical subspecialist[1]	$587,125
Registered nurse[2]	$88,006
Physical therapist[3]	$51,110
Respiratory therapist[4]	$3,447[5]

[1]Schloss et al. (2009).
[2]Jones (2008).
[3]Mercer, Szaniawski, and Guettler (2002).
[4]Stoller, Orens, and Kester (2001).
[5]This figure includes only training costs for the new respiratory therapist, not full turnover costs.

---

specialist. However, the actual turnover rate was about 5–8 percent (Schloss et al. 2009). While it is nothing to ignore, this rate is lower than the typical turnover rate for nurses, which is closer to 15 percent. A 2007 report by PricewaterhouseCoopers' Health Research Institute reported that the average *voluntary* turnover rate for first-year nurses was a startling 27 percent. (Note that this figure is the voluntary rate—the rate among people choosing to leave their job, not those being fired.) One-quarter of first-year nurses are leaving their jobs! While the cost of replacing a nurse may be much lower than that to replace a physician in an academic health center, the actual costs may not be much different because of the higher number of nurses who need to be replaced regularly. For example, PricewaterhouseCoopers (2007) reported an average of $300,000 per organization in nursing turnover costs for every **1 percent increase in turnover—not the total amount**. One can find similar data for other occupations, such as sonographers, who tend to have even higher turnover rates than do nurses.

Of course, we cannot attribute all turnover costs to stress. Turnover happens for any number of non-stress-related reasons, including promotions, retirement, or relocation because of a spouse's profession. We cannot eliminate turnover, nor would we necessarily want to do so. In some cases, turnover serves a purpose, such as in the case of an employee who doesn't fit the culture or is underperforming. Turnover can also be useful to manage the workforce size when demand weakens or the economy is not strong (i.e., use attrition to reduce the workforce rather than lay-offs or terminations).

However, we know that the relationship between stress (and especially burnout) and turnover is strong. Thus, while we cannot break down that $20 billion (which was already an estimate) and attribute a certain dollar amount to stress, we know that it is a high proportion of that figure. We cannot stop people from retiring, nor can we stop someone's spouse from accepting a job elsewhere. And we certainly wouldn't want to prevent promotions! What we can do, however, is prevent most stress-related turnover.

I can imagine a potential response to these arguments: *If employees can't hack it, why should we prevent their stress? Why not just find someone who can cope?* Unfortunately, some people have taken this thinking so far as to use an interview approach (called *stress interviewing*) that is intentionally stressful to test potential employees' responses to stress. It's a rational rebuttal, but it goes back to the main issues presented in the introduction: With so many people reporting stress, how do you find the ones who are not? Why push out an employee who could thrive if not for the simple everyday stressors that keep her from doing her job to the best of her ability?

The effect of stress on turnover and retention may be even more insidious than I have already described. In my research, I have found that there is a surprisingly large group of employees who would leave because of the stressful environment but, for whatever reason, are stuck in their job. I once heard an executive say something to the effect of, "Half my workforce has retired…Now I just wish they would leave." Because of the lower productivity these employees engender, their presence may be just as negative as the impact of the employees who left. This point supports my argument regarding the ineffectiveness of using stress to tease out the employees who aren't fit to work for us. In doing so, we will lose a good number of otherwise solid employees but retain certain employees whom we might prefer not to employ.

Health-Related Costs

Beyond turnover, there are other human resource costs associated with stress, particularly those more directly associated with health. Long-term disability claims resulting from stress and burnout are the fastest-growing type of claim in the United States and in much of Europe. In Canada alone, the number of burnout claims filed has gone up 500 percent while the number of claims filed for physical disabilities has decreased dramatically (Sabongui 2006). Again, these data represent all occupations, but there is nothing suggesting that they do not equally apply to healthcare professionals. The fact is that stress and burnout are increasing costs because people are filing more insurance claims.

A related issue is worker's compensation. Workers are filing worker's compensation claims for stress-related issues. Although there is valid legal debate on the legitimacy of such claims, they exist and may be something your organization will face. Even if direct claims of stress in the context of worker's compensation are disallowed, stress is associated with compensable claims for traditional workplace injuries (e.g., needlesticks and musculoskeletal damage), which means it still must be considered a worker's compensation risk.

In addition to insurance claims, the relationship between stress and health suggests a link between stress and sickness-related absence from work. Again, this issue is muddy and difficult to sort out. If you catch a cold, you will have difficulty attributing it directly to stress. Regardless, any human resources director will tell you that absences related to sickness have a significant cost. Obviously, such absences are not entirely preventable, especially in healthcare, where exposure to illness tends to be higher than in other industries solely because of the nature of the work. However, absences resulting from sickness that is indirectly related to stress should decrease if stress is addressed.

Organizational Consequences of Stress and Burnout

- Higher turnover
- Healthcare costs

THE IMPACT ON PATIENTS

So far, we have highlighted the costs (direct and indirect) associated with stress from the perspective of clinical staff, administrative staff, and, more generally, the organization as a whole. If you aren't convinced yet, try looking at the issue this way: Stress among your employees significantly affects the quality of care they provide to their patients. It leads to medical errors, near misses (most of which are not reported), and lower patient satisfaction.

Of course, some of these repercussions result from the turnover discussed earlier. An increasing body of evidence suggests that nurse turnover, staffing shortages, and related issues severely affect the quality of patient care. Such research is well established and familiar to most healthcare executives, so let's focus on the more direct impact that stress can have on patients.

For example, I recently published a study (Halbesleben and Rathert 2008) in which my colleague and I found that physician burnout was associated with patient outcomes (e.g., post-discharge recovery time) after accounting for variables, such as severity of illness. Clearly, the relationship is not a clean, directly causal one. We anticipate that the relationship is driven by such problems as poor communication about treatment plans between burned-out providers and their patients.

Obviously, some of the increase in recovery time may also be the result of medical errors. Earlier, I discussed the possibility that burnout is associated with medical errors because of an inability to invest the appropriate psychological and time resources on safety procedures. The links between burnout and patient safety have been growing and are startling. While we still cannot attach an exact figure to the number of avoidable medical errors attributable to stress and burnout, the literature supports the idea that there is a relationship between the two.

An offshoot of this idea is medical error reporting. Research suggests that burned-out healthcare professionals who are still willing to report medical errors likely see reporting as a necessary resource allocation, or at least realize that the costs of not reporting are simply too high (Halbesleben et al. 2008). However, emerging research suggests that they may be less likely to report near misses—that is, instances in which an error did not occur but likely would have if someone hadn't intervened. Near-miss reports are typically voluntary, in the sense that no one would know about these events if they weren't reported. As a result, healthcare professionals may see reporting as an extra part of the job and feel that resources should not be allocated for it. Near-miss reports present an extraordinary learning opportunity, but burnout seems to be keeping organizations from learning from them.

One of the more established patient consequences of burnout is lower patient satisfaction. This relationship has been the crux of most burnout outcomes research and is consistently replicated. There is a host of possible mediating factors, such as poor communication, that help to explain this relationship; however, burnout seems to be the point at which problems start.

As argued by Jean-Pierre Neveu (2008), some of the reductions in patient satisfaction are actually the result of mistreatment of patients by healthcare providers. While the focus of research has been in the opposite direction (patient abuse of professionals), there is some evidence that burned-out healthcare providers are more likely to treat patients abusively. While more research is needed on this serious issue, there is ample evidence to suggest a problem exists.

TAKEAWAY POINTS: THE COST OF STRESS AND BURNOUT TO HEALTHCARE

An absolute dollar figure cannot be placed on the cost of stress and burnout to the healthcare profession. There are too many variables involved and too many connections that have yet to be solidified. The impact of stress is too individualized, context sensitive, and time dependent to be pinned down to a firm figure.

Moreover, I recognize that although evidence clearly links stress with these serious outcomes, we will never be able to come up with absolute causal links between stress and the outcomes described in this chapter. Ethical issues aside, I doubt many healthcare organizations and their employees would be willing to volunteer for a randomized, controlled trial of stress and outcomes in which one group is randomly assigned to the "high stress group" and observed for such things as lower performance, injuries, turnover, insurance claims, and medical errors.

This impossibility, however, doesn't diminish the main message here: There is a *significant* long-term cost of stress among healthcare professionals. To summarize, here is the straightforward case for why you should be concerned about stress and burnout in your organization:

- Stress and burnout are associated with lower employee performance, turnover, and diminished health.
- As a result, stress and burnout represent significant financial costs to healthcare organizations.
- Stress and burnout also are associated with lower-quality care as a result of medical errors and lower patient satisfaction.
- Because burnout is largely preventable, the negative consequences it engenders are at least partially preventable as well.

The bottom line is that stress and burnout in healthcare organizations lead to considerable financial and human costs and **must be addressed**.

FURTHER READING

Garman, A. N., P. W. Corrigan, and S. Morris. 2002. "Staff Burnout and Patient Satisfaction: Evidence of Relationships at the Care Unit Level." *Journal of Occupational Health Psychology* 7 (3): 235–41.

Vahey, D. C., L. H. Aiken, D. M. Sloane, S. P. Clarke, and D. Vargas. 2004. "Nurse Burnout and Patient Satisfaction." *Medical Care* 24 (2): 57–66.

CHAPTER 2

Defining the Problem of Stress and Burnout in Healthcare Organizations

Every day when I come to work, it's just one more frustration after another. The harder I try to avoid problems, it seems the more likely I am to have problems. I'm just getting tired of putting so much into the job without getting anything back.

—Unit clerk at a community hospital

Frustrating
Frustrating
Stressful
Frustrating and stressful
    —Responses of four nurses in a community hospital intensive care unit when asked about the personal impact of making constant adjustments in work because of poor work design (and I could have listed at least 20 such responses)

HOW DID WE GET SO STRESSED OUT?

In this chapter, I am going to present a number of hypotheses about how we manage stress. Before dismissing these hypotheses as "just theory," bear with me. As researchers, we develop theories to make sense of our world. They help us organize our thinking about how things should work and why they should work that way. When we see a colleague lash out at a coworker, we may say, "Wow, he's having a really bad day," or, "Wow, he's an incredible jerk." We don't know for sure why the colleague lashed out. The reason could be some terrible combination of a jerk having a bad day, but we have developed our personal theory about why he acted that way.

We also develop theories so we can plan for the next situation. If we conclude that our colleague is having a bad day, we might cut him a little slack or wait until tomorrow to ask him a challenging question (or put off a terrible performance review centered on his interactions with colleagues). If we conclude that he's a jerk, we may avoid him altogether.

The point is that theories help us understand our world and recognize how we should act in future situations. In the case of stress, theories will help us understand why we are so stressed out, how we react to stressors, and why some people seem to deal with stress more easily than others do.

The Transaction Stress Model

One of the more influential theories about stress was proposed over 25 years ago by Richard Lazarus and Susan Folkman. Their theory is based on an individual's appraisal of his environment. When faced with something potentially stressful, individuals make two appraisals of their situation. In the first, called the *primary appraisal*, the person determines whether he has a stake in what is happening to him and whether it might hinder his personal goals (Lazarus and Folkman 1984). In other words, the individual tries to determine whether he is facing a stressor. For example, when a new patient is admitted to the intensive care unit, the staff members on the unit are faced with an additional demand. However, they may or may not perceive this demand as stress-inducing. If the unit is unusually busy that day, the new patient will require a high level of staff resources, and if they don't have a bed available for the patient, the new patient will likely be seen as a significant stressor. On the other hand, if relatively little is happening on the unit at the time, the new patient may be seen as a welcome break from boredom. At times, the same situation can be stressful or a minor blip on the radar, depending on such contextual factors as what else we are doing at the moment, what other demands we are facing, and who is around to help us.

If, in the first appraisal, the person determines that a stressor does exist (e.g., that extra patient is going to be a stressor), he makes a *second appraisal*: He considers whether he has the resources to cope with the stressor. Depending the outcome of this evaluation, the individual will determine how best to cope with the stressor. This determination is what enables some people to handle a stressful situation with relative ease. If members of that ICU staff are accustomed to busy days, bed shortages, and challenging patients, they may have structures in place that allow them to easily deal with the situation.

Lazarus and Folkman (1984) proposed that we cope with our stressors in a variety of ways. Two of these ways are active coping and avoidant coping. *Active coping* refers to the use of methods to manage a situation so as to regain control; *avoidant coping* refers to avoidance of the situations that cause stress. People are more likely to use active coping when their secondary appraisal suggests that they have the ability and resources to make changes that will improve the stressful situation. On the other hand, when people perceive that the situation cannot be changed or that they do not have the resources to initiate a change, they are more likely to use avoidant coping. You might think of this distinction in terms of "fight or flight." If we have the resources to fight, we do. If we don't have those resources, we run. While the transaction stress theory has been useful for over 25 years and is well supported by evidence, it still leaves us with some questions. The theory proposes that we assess whether we have the resources to deal with a situation, but it does not define resources or explain how we use our resources. To help address some of the questions left unanswered by the transaction stress theory, we turn to another stress theory that has attracted the attention of many researchers over the past 20 years: the conservation of resources theory.

Conservation of Resources Theory

Proposed by Stevan Hobfoll in 1988, the *conservation of resources theory* emphasizes the role of motivational resources, defined as objects, states, personal characteristics, and symbols that we value and that can be expended to gain additional resources. Hobfoll (1988) developed a list of common resources, which include a home (object), employment (state), self-esteem (personal characteristics), and money (symbols). Similarly to the transaction stress theory, the conservation of resources theory argues that the key is to understand our "resource account" from which we might draw and how we use those resources.

According to the theory, our stress results from one of three triggers. The first is a loss of resources. Loss of employment, for example, is a significant stressor for most people. This example is rather dramatic; there are other less significant resource losses that we experience. For example, when someone shows up late for an appointment, we have lost time waiting. A public reprimand may cause us to lose self-efficacy and status. Resignation of a close colleague may mean we have lost a valued relationship. The point is the same: If we draw on our pool of resources against our will, we experience stress.

The second trigger is the perception that our resources are threatened. For example, if we hear that our organization will be laying off employees because of economic conditions, we may experience significant stress even if we have not yet lost our job. This source of stress affected many people in the recent financial crisis, even though they hadn't lost their jobs and their homes' value had not necessarily changed. As a result of constant reminders from newscasters about the crisis, people developed the perception that they could lose their jobs even if their employers had not communicated layoff intentions.

The third trigger is situations in which the resource investments we have made are not producing gains. To acquire and protect resources, we typically need to invest them in other areas. For example, training to become a nurse requires an investment of time, money, and energy. However, that investment yields skills and employment opportunities (many, in fact, given current shortages in nursing). Once that training is completed, further investment of time and energy will be required for it to yield resources, such as money and job satisfaction. As we acquire resources, we put them to work to gain new and better resources. Sometimes, however, those investments don't work out as we had hoped, and the result is stress. If you spent years attaining a master's degree in health administration with the hopes of getting a promotion and it did not happen, you would likely experience stress.

This last trigger is crucial to our discussion of stress and strain at work. Later in this chapter, I will review some of the most common stressors faced by healthcare professionals (both clinical and administrative staff). Most of these stressors involve an inadequate return on resource investments. People invest a lot to become healthcare professionals and to do their jobs. While many think of healthcare jobs as noble professions, much of the work done in healthcare goes unrecognized. For many, it is a thankless job.

The resource investment process is also important because we use it to deal with the first two stress triggers (loss of resources and threat of loss). When we face resource loss (or threat of loss), we typically invest additional resources to minimize the loss. When we think we might lose our job, we invest time to update our resume, search for job openings, and tap our network for job opportunities. Thus, according to the conservation of resources theory, coping is an investment of resources. When we have a lot of resources, we engage in more active coping. When we don't have resources, we lean toward avoidant coping.

Conservation of Resources Theory

According to conservation of resources theory, our stress comes from three sources (with examples):

- Loss of resources, for example:
  - Job loss
  - Resignation of a close coworker
- Threat to resources, for example:
  - Media reports about job losses
  - Proposed changes to reimbursement
- Bad investment of resources, for example:
  - Working on a project but not receiving recognition for doing so
  - Helping a friend (or patient) but not receiving a reciprocal favor
  - Achieving a degree but not finding a job or getting a promotion

Understanding resource investment helps us understand how we go from experiencing stress to burning out. Recall from the Introduction that burnout is a response to extreme work stress. It is the point where we can't take any more stress, where we are exhausted. According to the conservation of resources theory, we reach a point where we keep investing resources to cope with stressors but don't get anything back to replenish the resources we've used. Eventually, we run out of resources; our account is empty. As we'll discuss in the next chapter, arrival at this juncture leads to a whole host of problems.

How We'll Use These Theories

So why have I spent so much page space on stress theories? Why don't I get to the meat of the issue and talk about what is causing stress in healthcare? The theories help us understand the stressors and why they are stressful, which in turn will hopefully help us design system-level changes to address them. The reality is, though, that healthcare professionals will still experience stress. Fifty years ago, doctors and nurses experienced stress. They may not have been dealing with complex issues of coordination of care and pay for performance, but they experienced stress nonetheless. Fifty years from now, we will have solved many of the problems I will describe in the next paragraphs, but new concerns will likely emerge. When they do, healthcare professionals will deal with them by using the same processes. They will assess whether the concerns are stressors, evaluate whether their resources match the demands placed on them, and invest some of those resources to deal with the stressors. An understanding of the specific stressors people face may be useful to have, but more important is the process they follow to deal with those stressors. While our context (and thus our stressors) will change, the psychological processes we use to cope with those stressors likely will not.

The theories are also useful because they give us direction for dealing with the stressors. If we know that stress results from issues with our resources, replacing those resources and building new resources probably will help to alleviate it. Later in the book, I will discuss the development of such solutions. For the moment, let's consider some of the common stressors healthcare professionals face.

STRESSORS AMONG CLINICAL STAFF

All clinical staffs regularly face a common list of stressors. While a complete list of these stressors is beyond the scope of this book (and likely could take up several volumes), a number of key stressors are worthy of mention, either because I have encountered them frequently in my discussions with healthcare professionals, because they are frequently discussed in the literature, or because they are much worse (or much less worse) than people realize.

Patient Demands

Perhaps the most obvious stressor faced by healthcare professionals is the demand placed on them by patients. The daily grind of meeting with patients, explaining diagnoses, devising and implementing treatment plans, and answering their questions requires some investment of resources. Remember, however, that healthcare professionals are trained to deal with these types of demands and usually are able to deal with even particularly difficult cases and patients. A report by Lise Fillion and Louise Saint-Laurent for the Canadian Health Services Research Foundation (2003) summarized this idea nicely when they wrote, "The main source of stress for [palliative care] nurses is not daily contact with people whose life is ending, but the fact they constantly must wage battle in a disorganized system so these people can spend their last days in dignity and respect for their personal values." In other words, for people working with a delicate patient population (people near the end of life), issues with the system in which they are trying to complete their work are causing the stress, not the patients.

In making this statement, I am not diminishing the emotional stress associated with caring for patients. Working with people takes an emotional toll on care providers, especially when they are expected to offer excellent service to people who may not be at their best or most chipper. The topic of emotional labor is well established in the literature, which suggests that defiance of internal states (e.g., acting nice when feeling angry) can be a significant source of stress. This topic applies both to direct work with the patient and interaction with the patient's family members. Working with patients clearly has an impact on healthcare professionals, but we're finding that this impact has diminished over the years and that issues related to the workplace context have become much more important.

Workload, Staffing, and Scheduling

For many healthcare professionals, issues of workload, staffing, and scheduling are significant, related sources of stress. In a systematic review of nursing stress literature, McVicar (2003) found that workload and inadequate staff cover were among the most common stressors for nurses. As a result of low staffing levels, professionals are more likely to work less desirable schedules and have a greater overall workload. Stordeur, D'Hoore, and Vandenberghe (2001) ranked high workload as the most significant nursing stressor in terms of the impact it has on nurses. These issues are not necessarily quickly resolved: Even if organizations had the resources (e.g., money, time) to address staffing, the pool of nurses seeking employment may not be large enough to meet their needs.

With regard to scheduling, the most stressful issues appear to be working overnight shifts and working mandatory overtime. The common theme between these issues is interference with other aspects of life. Working overnight shifts makes other social aspects of life difficult (in part because of sleep disturbance), and working mandatory overtime makes balancing work and nonwork life challenging because of a lack of predictability.

Working with Other Professionals

We all know that dealing with other people causes stress. In their study, Stordeur, D'Hoore, and Vandenberghe (2001) ranked conflict with other nurses and physicians as the second most significant stressor in terms of the negative impact it has on nurses. The high degrees of autonomy and professionalism in healthcare, as well as historical hierarchical structures, have made communication among healthcare professionals challenging.

Some of the concern about working with other professionals goes back to concerns about leadership. In his systematic review, McVicar (2003) found that leadership played a significant role in nursing stress. The study by Stordeur, D'Hoore, and Vandenberghe (2001) elaborates on this subject somewhat, noting that the transactional leadership style, which focuses on intervention as a means of correcting behavior (called *management by exception*), is perceived as a stressor by staff. This outcome is partially caused by how frontline managers are typically chosen; they are often chosen for their technical expertise (e.g., they are great nurses, physicians, or technicians) and not for their managerial or leadership skill. As a result, they focus on technical expertise and look for deviations from accepted practice rather than proactively address the work environment to make it better.

Working with Technology

As a result of the quality movement in healthcare, greater emphasis has been placed on using technology to improve quality and safety outcomes. However, emerging research on these technologies suggests that they are often implemented without fully considering the impact they have on the workflow of the employees using them. Technology that is often intended to make their jobs easier becomes a significant stressor for healthcare professionals because of the learning curve involved in navigating the new system. As the emerging study of workarounds in healthcare suggests, many professionals find ways of working around the technology to avoid the stress it causes them. In some cases, the workaround bypasses the safety gains that the technology was meant to provide. While there is less research on this topic than on some of the others we have discussed, healthcare administrators' interest in the subject will certainly grow as these technologies proliferate.

The stress associated with implementation of new technologies reflects a broader stressor among clinical staff: poorly designed work processes. Blocks in the work process resulting from poor system design are a significant source of frustration for healthcare professionals. The quotes that opened the chapter express this emotion. When we asked a group of physicians, nurses, and pharmacists about how they feel when they have to alter their work processes in response to poor work design, the near-universal answer was "frustrated." That they come up with their own solutions to how the work should be done highlights an issue from the Introduction that we will elaborate on later in the book: They know how to fix the problem. The employees have the solutions and are ready to implement them. However, if we don't capture their ideas in a systematic way, we end up with idiosyncratic solutions to the problem that make our healthcare processes unreliable.

STRESSORS AMONG ADMINISTRATIVE STAFF

In some ways, the stressors described in the previous paragraphs are also stressors for administrators. Stressors experienced by clinical staff will likely make their way to administration and become problems that administrators are left to address. Poor leadership is a stressor for administrative staff just as it is for clinical staff. Moreover, the stressors discussed earlier have other implications for administrators. For example, staffing shortages also affect administrators, who must fill positions and retain the staff they do have. They also try to manage the schedule in ways that optimize resources. Clearly, these issues can lead to stress. In addition to these issues, administrators have stressors of their own to contend with.

Coordination of the Clinical Function

Much of the coordination of the clinical function falls on administrators. As any administrator dealing with this issue knows, it is a stressful aspect of the job. Managing the intricacies of professional autonomy, personality differences, and different resource needs across professionals is a tremendous challenge.

In addition to actual coordination of the clinical function, administrators are also charged with making patients' care *appear* coordinated. In other words, while care may be coordinated in a computer system or among the clinical staff, it may appear disjointed from the perspective of the patient. Think of the times you have gone to the doctor and received a bill with six or seven different charges, when you thought you had undergone only a single simple procedure. The management of public perception is a notable stressor for many administrative staff members.

The Quality Movement

Reports from the Institute of Medicine over the past decade have put tremendous pressure on administrators to shore up the quality of the healthcare provided in their facilities. This charge has subjected administrators to the challenges of measuring and reporting quality indicators, meeting the needs of regulatory and accrediting bodies, and shifting the culture of the organization in a direction more focused on quality. The last task, cultural change, is one of the most difficult things for a leader to initiate. People are inherently risk-averse and change-avoidant; healthcare professionals are arguably even more risk-averse than average and typically demand evidence before they agree to support change initiatives.

The quality movement is also subjecting administrators to financial stress. As payers increasingly hold healthcare organizations accountable for medical errors (by not reimbursing for them), administrators are applying pressure to minimize their occurrence. As discussed in Chapter 1, their job is made more difficult because stress among clinical staff may reduce the likelihood that they will report near-miss information that would be helpful in error prevention initiatives.

Issues of coordination and quality can also intersect to create entirely new stressors. I've frequently observed this issue in the context of quality improvement training. For purposes of improving patient safety through better teamwork, many organizations have implemented crew resource management training programs. Ideally, these programs concurrently train clinical teams that work together so they can easily transfer what they have learned into practice. This design is rarely practical, however. For one, shutting down a unit so everyone can attend training may not be feasible. Further, physicians often will not commit to full-day training sessions of this nature. As a result, they may separately attend a shorter version of the training program that is not conducted at the same time as their colleagues' program. As another example, I've observed resident physicians trained in teamwork and communication skills default to the methods of attending physicians who had not received the same training.

The stressors discussed in the previous paragraphs are not an exhaustive list but only a sampling of the sources of stress healthcare professionals face. After stressors have been identified, the next challenge is to develop an understanding of how individuals cope with those stressors, as their coping patterns play a key role in whether that stress becomes burnout.

COPING WITH STRESS

Research evidence has been fairly clear regarding the consequences of using active or avoidant coping. Benefits (in terms of future psychological symptoms) were consistently found to result from the use of active coping, and negative consequences resulted from reliance on avoidance strategies. That is not to say that avoidant coping doesn't play a role in dealing with stress. Sometimes taking time to avoid the stressor may keep someone from acting in a rash manner and making the situation worse (e.g., lashing out at your boss over a minor stressor). Remember, however, that avoiding the stressor doesn't make it go away. It will be there when you come back to it. This inevitable outcome is part of the reason intervention strategies based on avoidance, discussed in more detail in a later chapter, don't work. You can take a one-week vacation to "get away from it all," but when you leave the beach, that crummy job will still be waiting for you (with the added benefit of a week's worth of piled-up work!).

Coping is a key link in the progression from stress to burnout. People who cope well with their stressors do not experience burnout. Those who don't cope well are more likely to reach that stage.

Coping with Stress

While there are a variety of ways to cope with stress, the most common distinction is between:

- Active coping—methods that are used to manage a situation so as to regain control, for example:
  - Talking with your supervisor
  - Developing an action plan for addressing workload
  - Proposing changes to work process

- Avoidant coping—avoidance of the situations that cause stress, for example:
  - Avoiding troublesome staff on the unit
  - Missing meetings in which difficult topics are likely to come up
  - Delegating decisions you should be making yourself

TAKEAWAY POINTS: MANAGING RESOURCES MEANS MANAGING STRESS

In this chapter, we discussed the main theories about stress management as well as some of the primary stressors facing clinical and administrative staff. The goal was to give you a framework for thinking about stress. The logic presented in this chapter suggests that if we manage our staffs' resources, in particular by providing the resources they need to face their everyday demands at work, we can significantly reduce the stress they face.

The following list includes key points covered in this chapter:

- Stress results when the demands of our job exceed the resources we have to deal with those demands.
- When we face a potential stressor, we cognitively evaluate whether we are actually facing a stressor and whether we can deal with it.
- Our stressors come from three primary processes: (1) loss of our resources, (2) threats to our resources, and (3) bad investment of our resources.
- Common stressors among clinical staff include patient demands, workload, scheduling, working with others, and working with technology.
- Common stressors among administrative staff (in addition to those just listed) include coordination and quality.
- Stress is exceedingly difficult to measure. There are a variety of imperfect ways to measure stress; you will need to determine what works best in your context.

The next chapter takes stress a step further. Before we discuss how to address stress, we need to examine what happens when stress becomes too much, a situation we call *burnout*.

CHAPTER 3

When Stress Becomes Burnout

I reached a point where I couldn't take it anymore. I just couldn't give any more to the job. I guess you could say I gave up, but it didn't seem like it was worth it anymore.

—A nursing home aide

I reached a point where I'd walk into the room and I wouldn't even acknowledge the patient. I'd ask the resident or nurse what was going on, look over the chart, and bark out an order. They [the patients] were a problem that needed solving, not people.

—An attending physician on a cardiac intensive care unit

THE EXPERIENCE OF BURNOUT

Burnout is a response to chronic work stress. While the manifestation of burnout has been the subject of considerable scholarly debate, this chapter focuses on the most common perceptions of the burnout experience. The following discussion builds on the traditional three-component conceptualization of burnout that dates back to the early 1980s and the work of Christina Maslach (1982). Her work focused on emotional exhaustion, disengagement, and reduced personal efficacy.

Exhaustion

Exhaustion is the feeling that you have depleted your resources. When people say they are emotionally drained or they don't have any more to give, they are experiencing exhaustion. One of my favorite ways to assess exhaustion is to ask the respondent to indicate the extent to which the following statement applies to him: "When I wake up in the morning, I already feel too tired to go to work." I think the feeling described in that statement is the essence of exhaustion (and burnout in general); the mere thought of work is tiring.

Exhaustion is typically considered the "core" of the burnout experience. This designation is based on two ideas. First, despite the considerable scholarly debate mentioned earlier, all notable conceptualizations of burnout include some aspect of exhaustion. Second, research suggests that this symptom of burnout tends to appear first and leads to the other two symptoms. Therefore, if you want to understand the burnout experience, you had better understand the nature of exhaustion.

While early conceptualizations of exhaustion focused on emotional exhaustion, they have since been expanded to include cognitive and physical exhaustion. In other words, an employee can be "fed up" with work (emotionally exhausted), not have the cognitive resources to think straight about work, or be physically worn out by his or her job.

Disengagement

Disengagement occurs when a healthcare professional starts to pull away from his or her work. This symptom has also been referred to as *depersonalization* (reflecting the idea that when disengaged, one might treat people as objects) and *cynicism*. Poor treatment of others, reduced voluntary activity at work, absenteeism, and even turnover are all manifestations of disengagement.

Disengagement is a way of coping with the excessive stress that led to exhaustion. People naturally pull away from jobs that wear them out. They have two choices in this situation: fight or flight. If employees have reached the point of exhaustion, however, they will realize that attempts at fighting are likely to be ineffective. Instead, they will try to distance themselves from the sources of stress.

Reduced Personal Efficacy

Employees experiencing the third symptom of burnout, *reduced personal efficacy*, believe their ability to perform their job has diminished. On the surface, this symptom seems like a natural reaction to the first two symptoms. If a job is wearing an employee out and she is pulling away from it, she might feel as though she is not as good at the job as she once was.

As part of the burnout concept, this symptom is somewhat controversial. While it was a part of Maslach's original conceptualization, most contemporary researchers no longer consider it a symptom of burnout. It's not that people react to stress differently than they once did, but that empirical research on the subject has tended to find that professional efficacy is better considered either a consequence of emotional exhaustion and disengagement or a parallel development. In other words, while professional efficacy is related to burnout, research has not confirmed that it is a component of burnout. For this reason, the rest of the book will focus on exhaustion and disengagement. Nevertheless, efficacy does play a role in the process and is a key element of job performance. Because people must feel capable of performance to be able to perform, efficacy is an important variable to consider.

THE BREAKING POINT

At what point does stress become burnout? The turning point between the two is actually not known. A few years ago, researchers in The

Netherlands tried to pinpoint it by comparing pencil-and-paper (i.e., survey) burnout assessment scores to psychiatrists' assessments, but the idea never took off. The work was valid enough, but the experience of stress varies so much from person to person that the researchers had difficulty determining clear turning points.

Others have used arbitrary points on burnout or stress scales (covered in the next chapter) to determine whether someone is burned out. For example, if someone scores an average of 4 out of 5 on a burnout scale, that person might be considered burned out. This approach is useful in that statements like "X percent of our workforce is burned out" can be drawn; however, it is based on the assumption that everyone responds the same way to survey questions, and the multitude of evidence suggests that this is not the case. Surveys are well known to include response biases.

Instead of trying to identify the turning point, a better objective might be to decide whether we need to pinpoint one at all. The terms *stress* and *strain* (which burnout represents) are engineering terms; a bridge experiences stress each time a car goes over it and experiences strain when it starts to crack. We don't wait until the bridge collapses to say it is strained. Moreover, there may be differences in the severity of strain. As a result, most researchers treat burnout as a variable rather than designate a point at which burnout occurs. Burnout is commonly referred to in a discrete sense (e.g., "I'm burned out"), but degrees are often added to it as well (e.g., "I'm *really* burned out"). In this book, burnout will be treated as a continuum, although discrete phrasing may be used in some cases for purposes of simplicity.

We recognize that everyone experiences stress, so why doesn't everyone experience burnout? A report on stress at work by the National Institute for Occupational Safety and Health (1999) indicated that about a quarter of workers reported that they were "often or very often" burned out at work. While they vary, survey responses about stress indicate that stress is a more common problem than burnout. A variety of factors might help explain why some people reach the breaking point of burnout and others do not. For simplicity, we'll break these factors down into personal factors and organizational factors.

Personal Factors

A variety of personality traits are associated with burnout. People with Type A personality (characterized by time sensitivity, irritability, and high achievement motivation) tend to experience burnout at higher rates. Interestingly, while the relationship between Type A personality and burnout is statistically significant, the more startling finding has to do with other outcomes of stress. Type As seem particularly prone to stress-related illnesses, especially coronary heart disease.

Another personality trait, neuroticism, is even more strongly related to burnout. Highly neurotic people experience higher levels of self-consciousness, anxiety, hostility, and vulnerability. They appear to have difficulty dealing with daily stressors in comparison to other people; stressors seem to have an unusually strong link to burnout in neurotic individuals.

While the data have not yet been published, my own preliminary research suggests that those who suffer from adult attention deficit hyperactivity disorder (ADHD) tend to experience higher levels of stress. ADHD also appears to be related to their ability to adequately cope with stressors.

On the other hand, people who have high hardiness (a combination of high involvement, sense of control, and openness to change) tend to be less likely to experience burnout.

Another personality factor that seems to work against burnout is extraversion. Extraverts are confident and active and seek stimulation and excitement. As a result, they often surround themselves with other people to get that stimulation and excitement. This ready source of social support has been shown to be a key factor in reducing the likelihood of experiencing burnout.

Relationship factors may also play a role. Research has long held that people with spouses or partners at home are less likely to experience burnout. In fact, people who are single experience burnout at higher rates than those who are divorced! Recent research has expanded on these findings, suggesting that employees whose spouse shares the same occupation (e.g., both are pharmacists) and/or workplace (e.g., both work in the same hospital) are less likely to experience burnout, probably because their spouse is in a better position to provide useful social support to help them cope with their stressors and thus avoid burnout. Social support might be one of the most important resources employers can provide to help employees deal with burnout.

Organizational Factors

In addition to personal variables, certain attributes of organizations reduce or encourage burnout. Some of these factors were discussed in Chapter 2 (e.g., workload, staffing, and scheduling). Here, the focus will be less on stressors and more on organizational factors that influence the relationship between the stressors and burnout.

Employee access to feedback is one organizational factor that reduces the negative impact of stressors. For example, if a nurse facing a high workload was given constructive feedback about how the job could be done more easily or how to manage the workload, the likelihood of the nurse's stress progressing to burnout would be reduced. Similarly, if a healthcare professional is given autonomy to address the heavy workload, he or she may feel greater control over the job, which will reduce stress and help prevent burnout.

In a recent study (Halbesleben 2006a), I found that constructive patient participation in care can reduce the negative impact of stressors on physicians. In studying patient–physician dyads, I found that when the patient participated in care (e.g., informed the physician about his or her needs, communicated expectations, asked questions), the physician was less likely to experience burnout. These findings support the social exchange model of burnout of Arnold Bakker and colleagues (2000), who proposed that, when working with patients, the healthcare provider typically invests more time and energy in the relationship than the patient does. (This claim is questionable when applied to healthcare providers, especially acute care providers, who often have little actual contact with patients.) Consider their proposal in this respect: Healthcare providers often ask, "How are you doing today?" but how often do patients return the sentiment (at least genuinely)? This lack of reciprocity contributes to burnout because it becomes a continuous source of frustration for the provider. It fits with the idea of bad investments discussed in the previous chapter; the provider keeps investing resources in the relationship but realizes little return.

We also know that some variables are not as linked to burnout as people think. For example, some studies attest that there is a relationship between gender and burnout, while others claim there is no association between the two. This discrepancy brings up two important issues. The first is causality. Gender does not *cause* burnout; one is not destined to be burned out because he is male or she is female. Instead, gender co-varies with other causes of burnout, such as work–family expectations, workload, and other gender-role factors.

The second issue is data consistency. While more studies seem to show that burnout rates are higher among women, plenty of studies show that men have higher burnout rates. This finding may also be linked to the occupations of the participants in the study. For many years, the emphasis in the burnout literature was on service industries (especially nursing and teaching) that tended to employ more women than men. Workers in these industries also tend to experience higher burnout rates because their jobs involve working with people. The bottom line is that gender is likely not associated with burnout at all, or if it is, it is a meager, spurious association that could be better explained by examining specific dynamics of work (e.g., workload).

A similar explanation exists for studies that have found relationships between age and organizational tenure. Those variables are already highly related to each other (as we stick around our organizations, we get older) and appear to be negatively associated with burnout. In other words, people who have longer tenure seem to experience lower burnout. But does our burnout really diminish over time? As we get used to the way things work, our stress may abate. As we gain experience, we may be assigned better projects. In both cases, the relationship between age/tenure and burnout is better explained by some other factor (e.g., maturation or work assignments) and not by age or tenure per se. Also important is retention. People who are highly burned out are more likely to leave their jobs (the ultimate form of disengagement). Thus, those who stay around and have longer tenure must experience less burnout.

The intent of the last two paragraphs is not to critique the research but to draw attention to a trap managers occasionally fall into in drawing such conclusions as, "Women are more burned out; I should develop a program for them," or "I need to target the young people." Those statements might be true, but not because they are women or young, but because of other factors: They aren't getting the support they need, their expectations of the job are not being fulfilled, or some other factor is affecting their work. When we develop interventions, we need to figure out what we can change—and gender and age are two things we obviously cannot change.

HOW STABLE IS BURNOUT?

If someone reports high burnout today, is that person likely to report high burnout again six months or a year from now? Empirical studies of burnout tend to find high correlations over time, but we have to be careful not to equate correlations over time with stability of the burnout experience. Correlations are drawn from a pattern of scores across individuals in a sample. If one person's burnout score is higher today than it was yesterday and others in the study follow the same pattern, a strong positive correlation would be made. Does the presence of a correlation mean their scores are stable? No. It means their burnout has increased over time. (Burnout scores are discussed in more depth in the next chapter.)

That said, there are ways to assess stability over time by making statistical corrections to the correlations. In doing so, studies have found relatively high consistency over time. They also have found that, in general, the time frame of the study is irrelevant; studies that have explored consistency over time frames of three months to five years have obtained similar results.

These findings suggest that the factors underlying burnout are consistent over time. If you have a poor leader today and the same poor leader is in place a year from now, why would you expect burnout to change? The findings also support the idea that avoidant coping is not effective in dealing with stress. If the underlying causes of burnout are stable, avoiding the stressors isn't going to make them go away.

TAKEAWAY POINTS: IDENTIFYING VICTIMS OF BURNOUT

Burnout is an important outcome of stress at work. High levels of persistent stress lead to burnout. Everyone experiences stress, but not everyone experiences burnout, so studies on burnout are primarily concerned with what causes stress to progress to burnout. The following points summarize the ground covered in this chapter:

- Chronic stress leads to burnout.
- Burnout is characterized by exhaustion, disengagement, and, in some cases, reduced personal efficacy.
- Personal factors, such as personality and relationships, can influence the connection between stress and burnout.
- Organizational factors, such as feedback and autonomy, can influence the relationship between stress and burnout.
- Burnout scores appear to be consistent over time, regardless of the time frame studied, suggesting that the underlying stressors leading to burnout are also consistent.

We are getting closer to the point where we can address stress and burnout among healthcare professionals. However, as with any intervention, such efforts must be supported with data; otherwise, the work will be misguided. The next chapter discusses the myriad ways of assessing stress and burnout in healthcare and provides the tools you will need to get a handle on the extent of the problem in your organization.

CHAPTER 4

Capturing Stress and Burnout

There are days that I feel already tired before I go to work.
—Item from the Oldenburg Burnout Inventory,
intended to measure exhaustion

ASSESSING STRESS AND BURNOUT is a tricky endeavor. Think about what you have read so far. How would *you* assess stress? Easy mechanisms for measuring stress and burnout are not always obvious. The question, "Are you stressed?" is an ineffective gauge. People might be inclined to bias their responses. They also may not know what it means to be stressed, or they may have their own idiosyncratic definition of stress (as you learned in previous chapters, everybody experiences stress differently).

Good data are needed to move forward with intervention efforts. If we don't know how much stress people are experiencing, or more important, their sources of stress, we will have a difficult time reducing it. Moreover, if we want to evaluate our intervention later, we'll need a consistent way to assess stress over time. This chapter introduces a variety of options for assessing stress and burnout, focusing on some of the more popular, feasible techniques for healthcare professionals.

ASSESSING STRESS

Historically, a checklist of common dramatic life events (e.g., marriage, divorce, new job, death in the family), called the *Social Readjustment Scale*, was most commonly used to assess stress (Holmes and Rahe 1967). Each event was given a numeric score (e.g., death of a spouse is 100; divorce is 73; vacation is 13). The higher a person's score, the more stress he or she was experiencing. The problem with this approach is twofold. First, stress theories argue that stress is experienced within a context. For example, a divorce may not be that stressful if it released someone from a bad relationship (the same could be said for losing a bad job). A death in the family could be a welcome end to a long, difficult struggle with cancer. Likewise, in some cases, the scale didn't differentiate between voluntary and involuntary stressors (e.g., initiating a divorce versus receiving notice that your spouse filed for divorce). For these reasons, someone can take on a new job, get married, or experience any number of other things and not seem stressed. Such events may have brought about welcome improvements to that person's previous plight.

Second, the focus of the scale was on major life events. In most cases, everyday hassles, not momentous occurrences, are more commonly reported as sources of stress. Perhaps the infusion pump isn't working correctly, or overtime has been made involuntary for the week because of a staff shortage. These types of issues were not reflected in the life events scale, yet they have a profound impact on employees' experience of stress and strain. In short, the scale lacked sensitivity; someone could have been experiencing high levels of stress at work, but because he did not check off any of the major events listed, he registered low on the stress scale.

Seeking more "objective" approaches to assessing stress, some have advocated the use of tests that take physiological measures of stress, ranging from heart rate to blood cortisol levels. These approaches are somewhat valuable, and there is a host of evidence to support their role in the stress process, but again, they have two drawbacks. For one, employers cannot subject employees to regular blood draws. Second, if the goal is to address the problem of stress in the workplace, the information gathered from physiological measures is of limited use in this regard. Managing stress through biofeedback would be a daunting process in an organization. The goal is to understand and address why employees have these physiological responses, not the responses themselves. In other words, knowing that an employee has high cortisol levels may be a reliable marker that he or she is stressed, but what is causing the high cortisol level to begin with? While useful in establishing critical links between stress and health, for most organizations, assessment of stress via physiological measures is not feasible.

A logical next response might be to go back to our theories and try to assess an employee's resources, akin to checking the balance of a bank account to assess wealth. However, this approach poses some problems as well. First, the potential list of resources is huge. While Hobfoll (1988) tried to provide a list of resources in his works, it is impossible to fully capture the complexity of resources. Any such list either will be too long to be viable for study or, like the life event checklists, will overlook important resources. Moreover, the rate at which those resources are being drained also needs to be assessed. The banking comparison applies here as well: An account balance is not useful information if there is a stack of bills that need to be paid but the total amount to be paid is not known.

A variety of measures have been created to try to assess the stressors relevant to healthcare professionals. Historically, the Nursing Stress Scale (NSS) has been predominant in the nursing literature (Gray-Toft and Anderson 1981). Widely used in research, this scale has been translated into a number of different languages (e.g., Spanish and Chinese). In essence, the NSS is a nursing-specific variant of the life event scale that measures stress according to the frequency of stressful events. Since its inception, it has been expanded to capture nine sources of stress in the nursing profession, along with the frequency of each source (see French et al. 2000). This scale has been commonly criticized for neglecting to take into account the coping resources available to the respondent. The applicability of the NSS to other occupations is also questionable.

An alternative approach is to capture the respondent's overall feeling of stress. Instead of focusing on resources, this approach builds the appraisal of demands into the assessment questions. Cohen, Kamarck, and Mermelstein's (1983) Perceived Stress Scale (PSS) is one example of a tool that takes this approach. The PSS and other similar scales are more ideal tools in that they are general enough to apply to most occupations and tend to return highly valid results (although so do the others discussed in the previous paragraphs, according to some researchers). The general nature of these scales' assessment questions, however, makes diagnosis of specific stressors difficult. For example, consider this question: "In the last month, how often have you felt that you were effectively coping with important changes occurring in your life?" Would responses to such a question help pinpoint what needs to be "fixed" to reduce stress in the workplace? Not likely.

The bottom line is that a good measure of stress has yet to be designed. The key is to understand whom you are assessing and what you are seeking to measure. If you are trying to get an overall feel for the level of stress in your facility, the PSS may help you gather the information you need to do so. If you want to diagnose specific stressors among professionals of a specific occupation (e.g., nursing), then a scale similar to the NSS would work better. If you know that people are stressed, but you want to see where you might develop more resources to address the stress, you might compare your situation to Hobfoll's list of resources. No matter what you choose, keep in mind that there is no perfect tool for measuring stress among healthcare professionals.

ASSESSING BURNOUT

Although somewhat easier to measure than stress, burnout is similarly difficult to assess. Traditionally, it has been measured using pencil-

and-paper surveys. The following paragraphs describe some of the options available, how they approach burnout, and their advantages and disadvantages. Many measures have been developed, but their use may be questionable if there is no evidence supporting their effectiveness. For brevity, the discussion focuses on methods that have produced reliable and valid results (i.e., their outcomes are consistent over time and across items, and they measure what they say they measure).

The Maslach Burnout Inventory

The most established burnout inventory is the Maslach Burnout Inventory (MBI). Created in the early 1980s by Christina Maslach and Susan Jackson (1981), it is by far the most commonly used measure in the burnout literature. It is based on Maslach's three-dimensional conceptualization of burnout, which includes subscales for emotional exhaustion, depersonalization (called *cynicism* in the most recent iteration), and reduced personal efficacy. This concept, last updated in 1996 by Schaufeli and colleagues, has been translated into a variety of languages and is now available in three versions: a traditional version for service providers, an "all-occupation" version that does not refer to specific clients or customers and can be applied to nearly any profession, and a version for educators.

The MBI asks the respondent to indicate the frequency with which a series of statements apply to him or her. Because of its popularity, a great deal of attention has been paid to testing the MBI's reliability and validity. It withstands these tests well; the three subscales emerge as distinct factors. Moreover, it adequately discriminates between burnout and other related measures (e.g., depression).

Despite its common use, the MBI has drawn some criticism. The usefulness of its personal efficacy scale is questionable, as it tends not to work as consistently as the other two dimensions. Because it is a commercial test, the MBI is also expensive to administer; organizations have to purchase it from CPP, the test's publisher (see www.cpp.com). As this book goes to press, the cost is about $1.50 per test. In a large health system, this expense could add up quickly.

The measure's construction poses yet another problem. All of the items are phrased in the same direction (the respondent's burnout score increases each time he or she answers a statement affirmatively). People may figure out this pattern and respond without really thinking about the statements. For example, when faced with long surveys, people may repeatedly select the same response (e.g., always select "1"), regardless of how they really feel. Or, they may read the first few questions, realize they are all about the same topic, and respond similarly to all questions on the inventory without really thinking about them.

The Oldenburg Burnout Inventory

To address the concerns about cost and structure, and recognizing the limitations of the personal efficacy scale, Eva Demerouti and colleagues (2002) developed the Oldenburg Burnout Inventory (OLBI), which assesses burnout on the basis of two dimensions: emotional exhaustion and disengagement. (The quote at the start of the chapter is a sample item from the exhaustion subscale of the OLBI.) It is free to use for noncommercial purposes (i.e., you are not selling the measure). It also addresses the structure issue by balancing positively and negatively worded items. In other words, the respondent cannot lapse into an answer pattern and must carefully consider each statement. Developed in German, the OLBI has been translated into many languages (and validated) and applies to any occupation; it does not specifically refer to working with customers or patients.

Structured similarly to the MBI, the OLBI includes 16 statements to which the subject must respond. Rather than focusing on the frequency with which the respondent experiences each item, the OLBI asks the respondent to indicate the extent to which he or she agrees with the statement. This type of scaling (strongly agree to strongly disagree) corresponds with many other measures, so it can be consistent when embedding it with other measures in a larger survey.

The reliability and validity of the OLBI have also been studied. Like the MBI, it holds up well. A number of studies have compared the OLBI directly to the MBI, finding sufficient conceptual overlap between their emotional exhaustion and depersonalization/disengagement measures.

The Shirom-Melamed Burnout Measure

The Shirom-Melamed measure focuses on exhaustion as the core of burnout and expands this component to include elements of emotional, cognitive, and physical exhaustion (Shirom and Melamed 2006). As such, it does not include a measure for disengagement. Like the OLBI, it is available free of charge (see www.tau.ac.il/~ashirom/research.htm), has been translated into a variety of languages, and, on the basis of supporting evidence, has initially shown to return valid assessments. Shirom and Melamed ask users to share their results with them, and keep this information in a database. This tool may be particularly useful if you are interested in the energetic aspects of burnout.

The Copenhagen Burnout Inventory

Developed by Kristensen and colleagues (2005), the Copenhagen Burnout Inventory—the newest of the burnout measures—expands the domain of burnout beyond work to include personal burnout, work-related burnout, and client-related burnout. Kristensen and colleagues structured their measure in this way to allow for greater customization to the respondent. In other words, if the respondent does not work with clients (or patients), he or she would not take the client portion of the survey. While Kristensen and colleagues have reported initial evidence validating the measure, this tool is relatively new and should be used with some caution.

The Staff Burnout Scale for Health Professionals

As its name suggests, the Staff Burnout Scale for Health Professionals (SBS-HP) was designed specifically for healthcare professionals (Jones 1980). The SBS-HP measures burnout on the basis of adverse cognitive, affective, behavioral, and psychophysical reactions. It includes 30 items, 10 of which are devised to detect fake responses (i.e., responses given solely to look like one is not experiencing burnout when he or she actually is). Jones (1980) called these 10 items a "lie scale."

Initial evidence has shown the SBS-HP to be reliable and valid, but it does not have the same track record as some of the measures discussed earlier. Moreover, its somewhat idiosyncratic treatment of burnout is inconsistent with much of the literature on the topic. While having a measure specifically applicable to healthcare professionals may be desirable, quality of measurement may be sacrificed by using this scale.

A General Comment on Measures of Burnout

Many of the burnout measures require respondents to complete 16 to 30 items. So as not to add to their already heavy workload, shorter tools may be developed that can more quickly assess burnout among healthcare professionals. In general, 30 items should not take more than a few minutes to complete.

TAKEAWAY POINTS: GATHERING THE DATA YOU NEED

While we have some good options for assessing stress and burnout, we don't have an easy, perfect solution. Here are two important points to take away from this chapter:

- Stress is exceedingly difficult to measure. There are a variety of imperfect ways to measure stress; the best tool for the job will depend on the context in which the stress is experienced.
- While measures of burnout are somewhat more consistent than measures of stress, there are important advantages and disadvantages to each. To select an appropriate measure, you will need to determine which dimensions of burnout you wish to assess (e.g., disengagement).

In the next chapter, we will explore solutions to the stress epidemic in healthcare by addressing existing burnout and discussing prevention of additional burnout.

CHAPTER 5

The BRIDGES Program: Reducing Burnout in Healthcare Professionals

If management knew how to do our jobs so well, why would they need to make changes to them all the time to make them "easier"? I know how to do my job, and if they bothered to ask, I'd tell them how I could do it better.

—Maintenance worker at a long-term care facility

Being part of the [stress management] implementation team has done more to reduce my own stress than anything else I have done. The thought that my work is making life better for others here is extremely fulfilling.

—Nurse working on a medical-surgical unit in an academic medical center

AT THIS POINT, let's take a moment to see where we are in our journey. We started by making the case for why you should address stress and burnout in your healthcare organization. We have defined stress and burnout and explained the dynamics underlying them. This discussion provided a basis from which to structure interventions. In the last chapter, we discussed tools for measuring stress and burnout that can help evaluate the extent of the problem and the success of an intervention.

This chapter introduces techniques for reducing stress and burnout. This discussion may seem like the crux of the book, but in fact, this chapter isn't the most important. Consider this analogy: Imagine you just had a heart attack. You will require intensive treatment, perhaps an angioplasty, to address the blockage. But does that procedure solve the problem? Upon discharge, will the physician say, "Come on in when you need to be fixed again"? Hopefully not; instead, you will be given advice on dietary and lifestyle changes that will help you sustain a healthy body. In terms of importance, this chapter is the angioplasty; its purpose is to clear out the problem. In the next chapter, we'll delve into more detail on the "lifestyle changes" that will help maintain a less stressful environment.

TARGETING THE INDIVIDUAL VERSUS TARGETING THE ENVIRONMENT: THE LIMITATIONS OF "TREATING" AN INDIVIDUAL

One of two main approaches can be taken when developing intervention programs to address burnout: We can try to treat the individual, or we can try to change the environment in which that individual works. The former is tempting. Everyone experiences stress differently, so why not try to customize interventions to address it?

Skills-Based Approaches to Treating the Individual

Many programs for treating individual stress have been developed. The aim of these programs is to help the employee build coping skills that will enable him or her to address the underlying stressors that are leading to burnout. These programs include training in a variety of topics, including time management skills, interpersonal and social skills, stress inoculation, and assertiveness. They are attractive because they seem to be a catch-all. No matter what the stressor, wouldn't time management address it at some level?

The evaluation of these programs has been mixed. These programs occasionally reduce burnout but seem to do so only by alleviating its emotional exhaustion component (perhaps because by the time the person has begun to disengage, these techniques are too little, too late). The larger issue is that these programs do little to address the stressors in the environment. Someone can learn to better manage his or her time, but that person still will have to deal with workplace stressors, such as workload and low staffing. As such, these programs do not address the underlying cause of the burnout and subsequently are ineffective at reducing burnout over the long term.

Moreover, many of these programs assume that employees have never thought to manage their time better or improve their assertiveness. In many cases, they may have wanted to try these techniques, but they simply didn't work in their situation. Time management goes only so far if employees have more to do than time in which to do it. Time management doesn't make tasks disappear. Similarly, if an employee tried to be assertive but the approach backfired (e.g., he or she spoke up to a physician in the operating room, only to be shot down immediately for doing so), he or she is not likely to benefit from the training.

Individual programs also fail to fully consider a common finding in the literature: Burnout tends to occur in pockets. There is an element of emotional contagion to burnout; often many people working in the same department or on the same unit are burned out. They aren't similarly affected because all of the managers who manage time poorly were coincidentally assigned to the same unit; just like other epidemics (e.g., many people falling ill after drinking from the same tainted water supply), this spread suggests that there must be some centralized cause affecting all the individuals in an area. This phenomenon suggests that a better approach would be to determine the common underlying stressor leading to burnout among these employees rather than treat them individually.

Take a Deep Breath

Alternatives to the skills-based individual approaches are vacationing, deep breathing, meditation, and even squeezable "stress balls." For most people, these solutions are not that helpful. At best, they might give someone an opportunity to think through his or her reaction to a stressor (e.g., catching one's breath and not snapping back at a yelling patient or otherwise making the situation worse). Some evidence suggests that these mechanisms (e.g., meditation) put our bodies in a better position to deal with stress. In other words, while we still experience stress, these techniques reduce the negativity of our physiological reaction. Overall, however, they are not effective solutions for addressing stress and burnout.

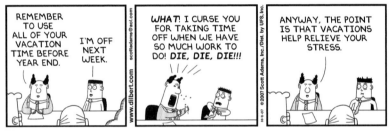

DILBERT: © Scott Adams/Dist. by United Feature Syndicate, Inc.

Why don't these techniques work? They don't work for the same reason avoidant coping doesn't work over the long run. When the vacation is over, the person returns to the same stressful environment and the same difficult boss or coworkers, not to mention a stack of work that has likely piled up over the last week in that person's absence. These mechanisms offer only a temporary reprieve. Further, many professionals are on call at all times. They receive calls and e-mail from work even while on vacation. They may be called in to fill in for someone else, or their vacation may be delayed as a result of mandatory overtime. Clearly, this approach is not an effective solution.

PROGRAMS FOR REDUCING BURNOUT

Programs that target changes to the stressful environment are far more successful in reducing stress than programs that focus on the individual. For example, Van Dierendonck and colleagues (1998) developed a group-based intervention program that focused on reducing burnout by adjusting employee expectations to match the work environment, which evidence showed to be effective in reducing burnout. Their program was based on the idea (a common one in healthcare) that employees' expectations about their jobs are often inordinately high and thus unfulfilled. This incongruity is part of the reason turnover is so high among early-career healthcare professionals.

Although such programs seem to be an attractive option, they are of limited usefulness in that they tend to seek universal solutions for organizational issues without taking into account the significant variety of stressors that may lead to burnout. Stressors prevalent in one organization (or in a department) may not exist in another organization. The Van Dierendonck intervention program was successful with its employee sample, but if misaligned expectations are not a problem in an organization (or not a stressor), such a program may not be that helpful. It could even make things worse; employees might start questioning the accuracy of their expectations when they are already appropriate.

As this discussion has shown, there is no catch-all solution to the burnout problem. However, there is a general *framework* for addressing stress and burnout, based on some of the ideas I presented in the Introduction: People want to be involved in the changes that happen in their jobs. Employees are the best source of ideas. If they are given an opportunity to share those ideas, they will be even more committed to seeing them through. All of these factors figure into a technique called action research.

ACTION RESEARCH AS A BURNOUT-REDUCING MECHANISM

Action research (sometimes called *participatory action research*) is an empirical and reflective process by which employees (in our case, healthcare professionals) work toward solutions to an organization's problems by focusing on the positive aspects of their experiences. It is widely accepted in organization development and management consulting and has experienced a significant resurgence in organizational theory and research. Rather than treating employees as a problem that needs to be solved, employees become the generator of solutions to the challenges at work.

I was introduced to action research a number of years ago while working on a consulting project with a federal fire department (see Halbesleben, Osburn, and Mumford 2006). The employees of the department were experiencing high levels of stress following the events of September 11, 2001. At the time, I had never used action research, but given my limited experience with the fire service, I was not in the best position to provide "expert recommendations." As I read more about action research, I became more convinced that it was the most appropriate strategy for the situation.

There are a variety of action research techniques. All are based on similar principles. First, the subjects of the research (employees) need to be **deeply embedded** in the process, not just "involved." Managers commonly pass out surveys or conduct formal or informal focus groups to gauge their employees' sentiments before designing interventions. For example, a manager might pass out a staff satisfaction survey, discover that the department's physicians are unhappy with staff policies regarding operating room scheduling, and make some changes to the operating room schedule. The subjects of the research are certainly involved in the process, but they are not deeply embedded in it. *Deeply embedded* means they helped design the survey and collect the data. It means they came up with the concerns *and* the solutions. It means they carried out the solutions (with their manager's support and resources). It means they were involved in evaluating the process downstream. Overall, it means the managers are giving up a lot of power for the good of all involved.

> In action research, subjects (or employees or stakeholders) are not just involved in the process; they are deeply embedded in it.

A second hallmark of action research programs is an action/reflection cycle, similar to Deming's Plan-Do-Study-Act (or Shewart's Plan-Do-Check-Act) quality improvement cycle. These cycles were an elaboration on the action/reflection concept, which involves trying different solutions to problems, reflecting on them, and then trying something different.

There are a variety of ways to engage in an action/reflection cycle. Exhibit 5.1 illustrates how the cycle might play out early in the process (before implementation of solutions). The idea is to hold initial meetings with stakeholders to elicit ideas about what is happening. These meetings are followed by reflection about the elicited ideas and integration with the evidence. For example, if social support seems to be a concern among your employees, you could look at the evidence regarding the best sources of social support and the best forms of support. Then, you could observe the work environment and engage employees in informal discussion. On the basis of these observations and discussions, you could elaborate on how support might play a role in the environment. After further reflection, you could conduct interviews with employees. After yet more reflection, you could conduct a survey and use quantitative data to elaborate further.

These sources of information or action are not set in stone; you can substitute whatever you feel is appropriate for the situation. Perhaps you can gather better information through focus groups. The point is that you are taking some action—in this case, collecting information—and then reflecting on how you might use that information.

Exhibit 5.1 Example of the Action/Reflection Process in Action Research

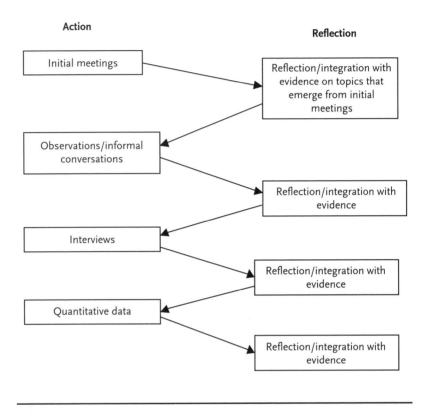

Beyond the deep embedding of stakeholders and the action/ reflection cycles, different action research programs part ways. Some offer steps to follow (e.g., Bruce and Wyman 1998). Over the next pages, I will propose a customizable framework that merges many of the ideas proposed in the action research literature. I have distilled these ideas into a model that seems to work best for addressing issues of stress and burnout in the workplace.

This framework is called BRIDGES, which stands for **B**uild **R**elationships; **I**dentify; **D**esign, **G**ive it a try, and **E**valuate; and **S**ustain. The acronym makes the program easier to remember. It is also symbolic. In 2001, the Institute of Medicine released *Crossing the Quality Chasm*. Arguably, one of the ways to bridge this chasm

Exhibit 5.2 The BRIDGES Action Research Framework for Addressing Stress and Burnout

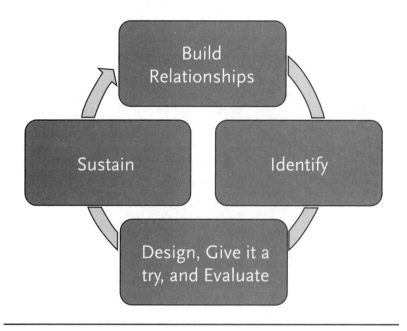

is to develop a workforce that is not burned out but engaged in providing safe, high-quality care. This program attempts to build that bridge.

More generally, it is central to the stress-strain metaphor. In Chapter 3, you learned that in engineering terms, stress is the momentary pressure placed on a structure (such as a bridge). When that structure starts to deteriorate, it is said to be strained. Further, the acronym refers the bridge you are going to build between your employees. A goal of this program is to help you develop a support network that will reduce the negative impact of stress. These "bridges" might be the most important structures you develop in your work.

The BRIDGES framework is a cycle of four steps (see Exhibit 5.2). The next few sections describe each step and how it can be implemented to reduce burnout in your organization.

Step 1: Build Relationships

Extensive efforts to build relationships must be made in action research programs. While better relationships are an *outcome* of action research, their development is also an important first step in the process. If you don't build strong relationships, your employees won't trust you enough to share their ideas. They won't feel as though you are willing to support their ideas. They will hesitate to take responsibility for implementing ideas because they will worry that they are being set up for failure.

Keep in mind how consulting projects usually work. Management brings in an outsider and tells everyone, "Here's the consultant; he's going to address our problems." We've all seen *Office Space*. Employees do not react favorably to consultants. They see them as people brought in to fire staff or tell them how they are underperforming in their jobs.

I've overcome this stigma in a variety of ways. While the fire-fighting project mentioned earlier is not a direct healthcare example, it is an example of an interesting approach to changing this perception. I did the obvious things, such as going out on calls with them, but what really made the difference was my effort to learn as much about the job as I could. I cooked. I watched football with them. I helped wash fire trucks. I even slept in the fire station for a few nights. I wore a uniform (just around the fire station, of course). These gestures broke down the barriers between us. They came to see me as a guy who was trying to learn as much about the job as he could so he could help them.

In healthcare, I make similar efforts. I don't just show up during the day shift when it's convenient for me. I stop by units in the middle of the night and on weekends. I engage in small talk and ask to see pictures of staff members' kids. I always explain why I am there and that I'm not trying to pester them. In general, I try to build a connection so they feel comfortable, and I try to find out what stresses them on the job by asking them to share some of their worst work experiences. My goal is to elicit great ideas about how their work experience could be better. The only way I'm going to achieve that goal is by showing them that they can safely share their thoughts with me.

My job is easier than a manager's in this regard because while I may be a stranger to these people, I don't have the baggage that comes with being part of management. For example, in some of the situations I have encountered, there is little trust in management because employees perceive that management is unwilling to make real changes. This mind-set can be a significant obstacle. Let's discuss some ways to address that problem.

First, managers need to be more visible. With all managers have going on, finding the time to chat with people can be difficult. Second, managers need to be sincere. People need to feel comfortable confiding in their manager and should want to work with him or her. Third, managers need to take an authentic interest in people's ideas. Small wins play a big role here.

Being more visible and sincere and taking people's ideas seriously are not new tactics. These ideas, packaged as a concept called *individualized consideration*, have been at the forefront of the leadership literature for years. Telling people to do these things is like telling people to lose weight. They want to lose weight and know what they need to do to lose weight (exercise and consume fewer calories), yet they can't manage to implement a plan of action. They simply don't make weight loss a priority. Similarly, to effectively reduce stress, you need to take this step seriously. The rest of this book is irrelevant if you don't build relationships. Let's explore these concepts in more detail.

Be Visible

Of the three tasks, this one is the easiest to implement. Start by carving out time **each day** to walk around your facility. Visit two units per day. Vary the times so you can hit multiple shifts (including the night shift—many interventions have derailed because the manager did not fully consider the implications for *all* staff, just those working during the day). On each unit, select at least one person and connect with him or her. Ask that person how his or her day is going, and ask a personal question (not too personal, of course) to find common ground. Then ask that person about what stresses him or her at work and what would make the job easier.

When chatting with staff members, be sensitive to what they are doing at the time. Remember, the goal is to reduce their stress, not make it worse. When I interviewed ICU nurses, for example, I tried not to catch them as they were walking quickly out of a patient room and to a computer. They were likely going to place an order or enter other information that they could forget. A more appropriate time might be when they are charting, but first ask whether they can chat for a moment when they are done with the chart they are completing.

Visits must become a habit—something done religiously every day. If you can visit units twice per day or visit more than two units, all the better. Eventually, people will recognize that you are with them in the trenches. You'll become aware of the stressors they experience daily. If you don't visit and chat with staff, you'll hear about only larger issues that have escalated to your suite, and by that point, the situation may be too difficult to turn around.

Be Sincere

When you visit units, don't be robotic and act like it's an obligation you need to get out of the way before you do "real work." A lot of my healthcare research has involved time-intensive interviews with busy people (e.g., ICU nurses). When I treated the interviews like just another to-do item on my list, I gathered worthless data; my questions were met with terse, short responses. When I started taking an interest in what the interviewees had to say, they trusted me and weren't afraid to share their thoughts. (I was studying medication errors—a topic people have difficulty discussing.) The resulting data were much richer.

Most important to remember is that an interviewer's genuineness is reflected in his or her responses to the interviewees' questions. When they ask about what you are doing and why, give them the best response you can. Don't just say something like, "Oh, I was just trying to see what it is like around here." Explain that you are making an effort to understand the stressors experienced in the facility to build the groundwork for change. Tell the interviewees about some of the great ideas you have heard, and ask what they think of them. Tell the interviewees some of your own ideas, and see whether they are still valid after the interviewees provide their feedback. When you put yourself in a position of vulnerability, you seem more genuine. Administrators often don't want to hear bad news (because they know they will have to do something about it) or good ideas (because they feel obligated to implement them). Keep in mind that in healthcare, where change is continuously proposed but rarely realized at the front lines, staff members are not expecting changes to occur overnight. Simply caring about their ideas will go a long way with them.

Take an Authentic Interest in People's Ideas

Not only must managers act genuine; they also must take an authentic interest in their staff's ideas. As with the previous concept, ask people for their ideas. Ask for feedback on the ideas you have collected. You demonstrate genuine interest when you flesh out the idea further with the person. Ask for clarification on details. How might the idea work? Who might be affected? Be careful not to play devil's advocate at this stage, however. Don't point out all of the idea's flaws and the ways it might not work. The time to assume this role will come later in the process, when ideas are vetted, tested, and evaluated. No matter how unrealistic or poor their ideas are, the goal at this point is to get staff to feel comfortable sharing them with you. When you react positively to abstract notions, you encourage people to share ideas that are less obvious and less "safe"—precursors to the development of innovative approaches.

Shoot for small wins here as well. Try a few of the easier and less controversial ideas. Implement them quickly to build momentum. Momentum is of utmost importance in these types of situations. While you certainly need to be thoughtful as you move forward, too much thinking can kill the momentum of interventions. Solutions can be refined throughout the process, so moving forward with some simple ideas is not overly risky.

Over time, these three steps will go a long way in building relationships. People will start to recognize that something is up. Someone cares about them. Someone is listening to their ideas and hoping they will share more of them. Let's move on now to step 2: identify.

Step 2: Identify

In this step, the relationships built in step 1 are leveraged to generate the ideas you need to solve the stress problem in your facility. Identification occurs in three phases: team identification, identification of challenges (in this case, stressors), and identification of opportunities to reduce burnout. This step goes by a variety of names in action research programs, but it is always included. Before changes can be made, you need to determine what the organization's problems are and the opportunities for change that are open to you.

Identify Your Team
On the basis of your visits and chats, identify employees who are particularly interested in the initiative. They may be important resources as you move forward. Any cause needs champions. As you identify your team, keep the following points in mind:

- Don't default to other people in management. Remember that there is a difference between leadership and management; you need leaders, not managers. You want the people whom employees go to when they have questions and concerns, who naturally engage others, and whom others listen to when things get hairy. You'll find that, in many cases, these people are not in management positions.

- Don't include those too high in the ranks, either. My wife worked for an organization whose executive director appointed himself to every committee. Not surprisingly, nearly every decision made on those committees defaulted to his wishes. Remember that you want this team to help you generate ideas on how to reduce stress; you don't want the meetings themselves to be stressful. Certainly get top management support and buy-in but explain that they will need to give up some control in the process. Clarify that the team will not be running every idea past higher management. Team members will become frustrated quickly if the CEO has to approve every suggestion they make.

- If there are unions in the organization, make sure they are involved. Union involvement can be tricky, particularly in facilities in which there has been historical infighting between them and management. Your ideas will not go far, however, if they contradict the collective bargaining agreement. Position the issue as a classic integrative bargaining situation: Addressing this situation helps both management and the union.

- Make sure you have good representation from all areas of the facility. Include physicians, nurses, therapists, technicians, pharmacists, custodians, and anyone else who may be affected by stress and burnout. Also involve key external stakeholders (e.g., temporary help agencies). Make sure all units are represented; you are going to need all the help you can get to generate ideas and implement solutions. You can always break into subgroups to work on specific aspects of the project (e.g., testing an idea, collecting evaluation data).

- Where should you house the team? Because the team will comprise a coalition of employees from across the organization, it needs to be protected from typical bureaucratic structures. For this reason, the team probably should not be part of the human resources (HR) department, even though much of the team's objective is HR's domain. The HR reporting structure is too clear, and in many organizations, the human resources department is perceived as an administrative group with no real decision-making power. Ideally, the team's reporting structure should be outside the organization's traditional hierarchy, similar to that of entities such as the office of clinical effectiveness (OCE) or the institutional review board. Given the impact of stress and burnout on quality of care, you might consider embedding this team in your facility's OCE. The efficacy of this approach will depend on the organization's perception of the OCE. At some organizations, the OCE is considered an intrusive organization that dictates how work should be done. If such a perception exists, the stress management team will have difficulty gaining traction, and you might be better off setting it up as a separate department or committee, even if it is a "virtual" committee (e.g., it doesn't have a definite office or staff).

Identify Challenges

My experience cooking and cleaning with the firefighters and sleeping in the firehouse did more than build relationships. Only through firsthand experience can one understand the stress firefighters experience when they are jolted out of bed at 2:00 a.m. to the sound of a buzzer and call assignments. My involvement was a perfect opportunity to identify stressors in the firehouse.

In the same way, many of the steps you will take in building relationships also will help you identify challenges. Even when you can't find anyone to talk to on a unit because everyone is too busy, you can glean a quick lesson from the stress they are experiencing. On the simple form in Appendix B, you can record observations and compile the data you collect while building relationships and then use this information to identify challenges. Complete the form after you finish your rounds; employees become paranoid when managers fill out forms while watching them work.

The process of identifying challenges and opportunities will be the first application of the action/reflection cycle discussed earlier. Information should be collected and integrated (with previous evidence on the topic and with the previously collected information) in a repetitive cycle. The following paragraphs describe how that cycle might play out in an organization. Remember that this approach is customizable; the survey example that follows may not be effective in an organization that is "surveyed-out."

The first task is to develop a list of potential challenges in the organization. However, note that I use the term *challenges*, not *stressors*. Challenges (e.g., regulatory updates) might present difficulties in addressing stressors. These challenges need to be understood to identify opportunities later. In some cases, there may be reasons why a challenge (and subsequent stressor) exists. For example, while barcode medication administration systems add steps to the medication administration process, those additional steps enhance the safety of the system. Instead of removing those steps, staff can be trained to use the system effectively so it does not impose such a burden.

It is also important to frame the stressors as challenges. Research (e.g., LePine, Podsakoff, and LePine 2005) suggests that stressors can be considered challenges or hindrances depending on one's perspective and the resources available to address the stressor. Framing the stressors as challenges implies that they can be addressed. Stressors are often perceived as problems outside one's control. Challenges, on the other hand, are seen as tasks that can (and even must) be resolved.

To identify challenges, begin with the informal observations you made while walking around your facility. From those observations, you should have an initial idea of what stressors exist in your organization. Once you have that information, work with your team to integrate it. Schedule a meeting, and put the information on a whiteboard. Look for themes. Don't worry if they are unrefined at the moment. The goal is to form a general idea about what is happening in the organization so you know what to ask about next.

Next, work with your team to decide what further information you need and how you can best collect it. Don't limit your options, and don't worry about consistency across the facility. For example, you might find a quick closed-ended survey works well for physicians (open-ended questions don't work with physicians), while detailed interviews or focus groups work well with nurses. Open-ended surveys have shown to be effective for pharmacists.

Further, don't limit yourself to one mode of data collection per group. After each data collection, integrate the information, determine what you have learned, and tailor the next data collection to dig deeper. For example, if your surveys indicate that people perceive a lack of management support, you could use interviews to follow up and find out more about this topic.

Some of the data collection techniques are better suited for certain purposes. Surveys are useful for identifying stressors, determining levels of burnout, and breaking down the data by demographics (e.g., occupation, unit), but they are not well suited for identifying opportunities to reduce stress and burnout. Focus groups are good for discussing ideas, but the quantity of information you can collect will be limited because you will have to juggle the perspectives of many people at the same time, and some people may not want to share all of their ideas in public. (See Appendix B for tips on running more effective focus groups.) Your team can coordinate these decisions so you maximize the data you gather from each collection.

These tasks should be delegated to team members. You will find that employees are typically more comfortable talking with their peers than with a supervisor (otherwise, they would have already talked to you!). Don't take them on alone; you'll just create stress for yourself.

Identify Opportunities

As you collect information about challenges, think about (and collect information about) potential solutions. Some solutions will develop naturally. In addition to providing information about stressors, interviewees often volunteer potential fixes for the problem. Data collection is more effective when it is structured around solutions. For focus groups in particular, ground rules should be set up front. The most important of these rules is to require that anyone venting a concern also offer at least one way to address it. Compliance with this rule will ensure that the focus group doesn't dissolve into a "howling session" and will steer the group toward coming up with challenges that have solutions.

When using interviews or focus groups to generate solutions, thoroughly flesh out the participants' ideas. If someone comes up with a solution (e.g., more nurses are needed), work through how it might be implemented. Focus groups are good for this purpose because participants can bounce ideas off each other and you can immediately observe their reactions to those ideas.

On the downside, a focus group can get out of hand when it is running with an idea. The group may become overly excited about a solution and expect it to be implemented, only to become upset if it isn't. On the flipside, participants may shoot down each other's ideas prematurely and thus discourage further ideas from coming to the fore. These problems can be largely prevented by establishing clear ground rules and goals up front. Clarify that you are developing ideas that may not be implemented long term. Remind the group that ideas can be tested and need not be dismissed right away. You can set expectations without being negative about the process.

The person (or better, persons) running the focus group also can manage these issues. If someone consistently shoots down ideas, encourage that person to provide a solution that will work. If the group develops unrealistic expectations about implementation and immediate impact, play devil's advocate (not too much—just enough to bring the group back to earth).

The processes of identifying your team, challenges, and opportunities will be long. They will not proceed quickly—and shouldn't. Ideas should have time to gel. Ideally, these tasks should take at least six months so you can build momentum, integrate ideas, and give people plenty of time to think of new solutions after the focus groups. Once you have some initial ideas about the main challenges and opportunities in the organization, you can start doing something about them. Remember that the process of generating solutions is constant. People can come up with solutions well after you have designed and implemented earlier ones. In fact, if a solution is working but someone proposes another that might work even better, the initiative is achieving early success.

Step 3: Design, Give It a Try, and Evaluate

In this step, you use the data you have collected to design interventions, test them, and evaluate their effectiveness. As in step 2, you will need to rely heavily on your team in these efforts.

Interventions do not come prepackaged. To work, they must be based on the challenges and opportunities identified in the previous step. As discussed earlier in the chapter, the development and use of prepackaged interventions brought about the downfall of previous programs because they don't always work. These steps are a framework that can be tailored to your situation, not an exact solution to your problems.

For example, let's say that one of the common challenges was with technology—specifically that employees feel it adds more work when it is supposed to make their lives easier. Suppose an employee suggested designating "super-users" of the technology to assist other employees. *Super-users* are employees with additional training in the technology who serve as go-to people for employees working with it. They are peers of those needing assistance, not information technology employees. The literature suggests that they can play an important role in shaping the attitudes and behaviors of employees regarding new technologies (see, for example, Halbesleben and colleagues [2009]) and that they may reduce some of the stress associated with implementing new technologies.

On the basis of this idea, you could select a group of super-users (see Boffa and Pawola [2006] for ideas on how best to select these people), train them, and allow them to work with technology users for some period. Depending on the nature of the intervention, this period could be a few months or even a year. When the period has ended, you would review the initiative with all employees using the technology. You could use the same techniques described earlier: surveys, interviews, and so on. On the basis of the information you collect, you can evaluate whether the system is working and, if so, determine how it could be tweaked to work better. For example, you might find that the super-user program is working great and no changes are needed, or that it works but you need more super-users. Or, you might find that the super-users aren't helping much because the technology is so poorly designed that even support from a super-user can't make it easier to navigate.

In this example, we have taken an idea (super-users), designed a program around it, given it a try, and evaluated it. These tasks should be repeated for every intervention you implement, no matter how big or small. Again, this step takes you through the action/reflection cycle. You try new ideas, reflect on how they worked, and then try something else.

The evaluation portion of step 3 is especially important. Too many organizational interventions are developed and implemented but not properly evaluated. Change is not the same as improvement. As a result of unforeseen circumstances, an intervention could make the situation worse. Computerized physician order entry (CPOE) is one example of a technological intervention that has not worked as planned. While it was supposed to streamline the process, make it easier for all involved, and improve patient safety, a host of unintended negative consequences have been unearthed that have put many of the systems on hold or sent them back to the drawing board for more careful study.

So how do we best proceed with evaluation? Use the tools that you used to collect the data initially. If you conducted a survey to collect information, rerun the survey and examine how the results have changed. By using the same tool, you gather consistent measures over time.

Think carefully about the questions you are asking. Too often, organizations rely on "happy sheets" to evaluate interventions. In other words, they simply ask whether the person liked the change and do not consider whether it was effective. This problem has been prevalent in evaluations of crew resource management (CRM) training programs. CRM programs use aviation principles to train healthcare professionals on issues of teamwork and communication for purposes of improving patient safety. Often, however, these programs are evaluated on the basis of questions about whether the participants liked the training and whether they might use it in their jobs. Typically, they say it was great and that they will use it most of the time, but when observed later on the job, few are actually using the principles they learned. Happy-sheet evaluations do not reflect reality.

To evaluate your stress management program accurately, don't just ask participants whether they liked the program. Ask whether their stress has been reduced as a result of the program (the outcome), whether they feel they are receiving more support—or whatever the target of the intervention was. These questions will prompt them to furnish the information you need to move forward.

Evaluation is critical.
Change is not the same as improvement.

When you have finished with step 3, you should have implemented a process that will have the greatest impact on reducing stress in your organization. The next step is to sustain the effect of this process.

Step 4: Sustain

Sustainability has become a buzzword over the past few years. One of the keys to action research is development of a culture that addresses issues as they come up rather than allowing them to become more significant long-term problems. Your stress management program will be worthless if the same (or new) stressors creep up a few months down the road—and they will if you don't establish structures to address them as they arise. Think about the stressors healthcare professionals dealt with ten years ago. Were they the same stressors we hear about today? Some of them are the same, but many new stressors, particularly related to new technologies, have emerged. Even if you addressed all the stressors in existence ten years ago, you will be dealing with new stressors today.

How can we sustain our work so that we don't run into future stress-related problems? The short answer is: Close the loop. Continue to make rounds of your facility on a regular basis, indefinitely. Not only do rounds enable you to monitor stress symptoms among your staff on a continuous basis; they also are simply a good management practice. (Quint Studer [2004] has written extensively about this topic in his book *Hardwiring Excellence*).

You also need to retain your team of stress management champions. People will join and leave the team, but the basic framework should stay in place. They can continue to come up with ideas for addressing stress and help test them. They can also help identify potential stressors in their own units and serve as critical communication channels to you. While your meetings will likely become less frequent and less intense, they should continue in order to maintain the structure of the stress management team.

The idea is to continue to build on your momentum. You may ride the momentum for a little while, but new stressors will certainly develop. If you have these basic structures in place, they will be easy to address. If you do not and have to restart the program, the road to recovery from even the smallest stressors will be long.

TAKEAWAY POINTS: TOOLS FOR REDUCING BURNOUT

In this chapter, we discussed how to address the burnout that already exists in your facility. Here are four main points to take away from this chapter:

- Dealing with employees on an individual basis by enrolling them in time management programs or giving them vacation time will have little long-term value in addressing concerns with burnout in the workplace. The environmental stressors will still exist.
- Similarly, one-size-fits-all programs typically are not successful because they do not account for the unique stressors of each organization.
- Action research provides a customizable framework for addressing stress in healthcare facilities.
- The BRIDGES program involves a cycle of activities structured around
    - building relationships with stakeholders so they are willing to work with you to address the stressors they face;
    - identifying a team to help you manage stress, the challenges your staff faces, and opportunities for reducing burnout;
    - designing interventions, giving them a try, and evaluating them; and
    - sustaining the change over the long term by continuing to cycle through the process.

The next chapter elaborates on the final step in the framework, sustainability, by discussing preventive measures you can take to address long-term stress.

CHAPTER 6

Taking Sustainability to the Next Level: Developing a "Stress-Free Environment"

You will work with patients who are at the lowest point of their lives and in extraordinary pain. Many will not be able to thank you for what you do. And yet, if even one does thank you, it will stick with you for the rest of your career.

—Emergency department nurse describing what she would tell a new nurse starting on the unit

I work here solely because of my coworkers. Without their support, I would have long since moved into a different career.

—Sonographer with 14 years of experience

THE GOAL OF Chapter 5 was to provide you with a means of addressing the immediate symptoms of stress and burnout in your facility. It also emphasized the importance of making longer-term "lifestyle" changes in the workplace to prevent recurrences. This chapter elaborates on *sustainability*—the component of the action research process that promotes lasting change.

THE ROLE OF PREVENTION

Before launching into the following discussion of solutions, take a moment to frame the issue of prevention. Every stressor in the workplace cannot be prevented (and shouldn't be; remember that stress in low levels generates the arousal we need to do our jobs). My experience with a large kidney stone a couple of years ago is analogous to stress prevention. After treating it, my urologist gave me a list of steps I could take to help prevent future stones. He then informed me that even if I took all of the steps, there was still about a 50 percent chance that I would develop another stone.

The idea is the same with stress and burnout. You can do only so much. However, if you have developed the process outlined in the previous chapter and take a few additional steps, the likelihood that stress will become a major problem will significantly decrease.

DEVELOPMENT OF A SUPPORTIVE WORK ENVIRONMENT

One of the most important steps you can take in addressing stress long term is to develop a supportive work environment. The literature has consistently shown that social support plays a critical role in reducing burnout. In this context, *social support* means a perception among employees that someone is on their side and willing to provide help when they need it.

Sources of Support

A few years ago, I conducted a meta-analysis of sources of social support and their relationship with burnout (see Halbesleben 2006b). A *meta-analysis* is a research project that combines all existing studies of a topic into one "big" analysis. By combining studies, you significantly increase the sample size of the research. This larger sample better represents the population and enables you to address broad questions of interest to many researchers. The purpose of my meta-analysis was to determine whether some sources of support (e.g., supervisors) are more valuable than others (e.g., family, friends) in addressing burnout.

My study revealed that work-related sources of support (e.g., supervisors, coworkers) had nearly twice as much impact in reducing burnout as non-work sources of support. That is not to say that non-work support isn't helpful; support from friends and family can be helpful when you have a bad day or are swamped with work. However, if you really want to address burnout, you need to develop support networks among the people in the workplace.

Types of Support

Why are work-related sources of support so much more valuable? The answer to that question lies in the type of support they are able to provide. Just as there are two forms of coping—active and avoidant—there are two forms of social support—instrumental and emotional. *Instrumental support* is tangible, practical support. For example, if you were having a difficult time creating a chart in PowerPoint, a colleague could show instrumental support by either creating it for you or showing you how to create the chart. (The former is obviously less helpful in that you will be in the same position the next time you attempt to create a chart.) *Emotional support* helps you feel better, but not necessarily by changing the situation. Again, if you were having a hard time creating a chart, your colleague would be showing emotional support if he empathized with you and said, "I feel for you. I've had that problem, too." You would take comfort in knowing that others have experienced the same problem, but emotional support won't actually help you with your chart.

As you might have guessed, instrumental support reduces burnout more effectively than emotional support does. It is better because it addresses the underlying problem; it eliminates the stressor more quickly. Again, that is not to say that emotional support is not helpful. Knowing that someone cares for us is important to our overall well-being. Some people may be able to come up with a solution just by talking about their problem with someone, even though that person can offer only emotional support.

On the same note, instrumental support may not always be the ticket to finding a solution. We all know people who are too quick to give advice, to the point where we want to avoid them, even if they are often right. Moreover, as mentioned earlier, if someone else deals with the stressor (e.g., your assistant creates the PowerPoint chart for you), you will just encounter the same stressor the next time around. In this way, instrumental support can enable bad behaviors. Finally, some people provide so much instrumental support to others that they have a difficult time completing their own jobs.

Thus, my meta-analysis found that work-related sources of support are more valuable than non-work sources in dealing with burnout. Supervisors and coworkers are usually in a better position to provide the tangible, *direct*, instrumental support that is more effective in reducing burnout, whereas family and friends are in a better position to provide emotional, *indirect* support—the less valuable of the two.

Developing a Supportive Environment

The results of the meta-analysis suggest that to develop a supportive work environment, we need to focus on work-related sources of support and providing positive forms of instrumental support. How do we accomplish such goals?

Encouraging and rewarding supportive behavior are critical in developing a supportive environment. One of my favorite scholarly articles is called "On the Folly of Rewarding A, While Hoping for B" by Steven Kerr. It's a brilliant article about how we tend to hope something will happen, while we reward (and thus provide incentive for) the opposite. Think about supportive behavior in the context of this idea. We hope that people will help each other, but we (1) don't provide them with the time to do so or (2) don't directly reward people for helping others do their work or, even worse, (3) "punish" people for helping others—for example, we overload them with so much work that if they do help others, they won't be able to complete their own work on time. As a result, they don't bother to help anyone else.

To develop a culture of support, leaders need to make helping and teamwork organizational values. If they clearly communicate that support is a valued behavior, it will be far more likely to occur in the organization. Support can be made a valued behavior through a variety of means.

First, evaluations and rewards should be based on support. Support should be part of employee performance appraisals, and regular feedback should be given on supportive behaviors. If employees are reminded every few months that their support is considered part of their overall performance, such behaviors will become more salient.

Particularly supportive behaviors should be publicly recognized with additional rewards. These rewards don't have to be financial; simple verbal appreciation will suffice. A management program doesn't have to be implemented for this purpose, either. Peer recognition of support is far more meaningful and sets the stage for reciprocation.

Second, employees need to be granted time to support each other. Lack of time is a significant barrier to engagement in supportive behaviors. Workloads should be structured in such a way that employees can get away from their jobs long enough to help someone without negatively affecting their own performance.

Another, arguably less orthodox, way to develop support is to hire spouses and partners. As discussed in Chapter 3, when spouses/partners work together, they are able to provide more support (and thus experience less burnout). When you work with your spouse or partner, he or she is both a friend and a coworker. Thus, he or she can provide both instrumental and emotional support— the best of both worlds.

Evidence suggests that such relationships are common in healthcare. Organizations that hire couples have a built-in support system for each employee in the relationship. Retention may also increase if the employees are both happy in the organization and become embedded in the organization and community over time.

Obviously, this proposition is complex. There must be a job opening for the spouse, and he or she must be qualified for it. In some states, marital status is a protected class; as such, you cannot consider it when you make decisions regarding employment. If the process is not managed appropriately, romance in the workplace and nepotism may become problems. If one partner leaves, the likelihood that the other one will also leave increases significantly. With all of these factors involved, an HR strategy for the hiring of spouses and partners is likely to have limited effectiveness. However, when the opportunity presents itself, the literature suggests that this strategy may yield benefits.

MANAGEMENT OF EXPECTATIONS

Unmet expectations are one of the most common instigators of burnout. This problem is a significant contributor to early-career health professional turnover, especially among nurses. The industry is seeing a great number of early-career nurses migrating to other positions or even out of the field because the job is simply not what they had envisioned.

To some extent, this issue needs to be addressed through education. More programs are approaching this problem indirectly (e.g., through interdisciplinary programs that work to improve communication between the various health professions). Other steps can be taken as well that will help align employees' expectations with the stressors expected to emerge on the job.

The first step can be taken before prospects even apply for a job. Realistic job previews (RJPs), a well-established HR management technique, provide realistic information about a position before the prospective employee even applies. The crummy working hours, difficult patients and family members, high levels of occupational injury, and so forth are all spelled out up front. In earlier iterations, RJPs were paper documents and included with paper applications. Today, most RJPs are provided online after candidates submit their application. Some companies even have potential applicants mirror an employee for a day so they can see what working there would be like.

The evidence suggests that RJPs work. For one, they increase commitment. If an employee decides to apply for (and later take) a job even though she knew it was going to be bad, she likely will be committed to it and will stick with it even through tough times. By recognizing the potential stressors of a job before taking it, employees are far less likely to experience burnout when the stressors do crop up. They will be prepared for them to happen and will have had time to gather the resources necessary to meet the demands.

Healthcare organizations have been hesitant to use RJPs, probably because recruiting is so competitive that they feel they can't afford to have prospects turn away. Simply hiring "warm bodies" to fill positions will just cause problems down the road, however. If there is a poor fit between the person and the job, he or she will probably become unhappy and stressed and then quit, and the position will have to be refilled. On top of that, given that burnout in organizations is emotionally contagious, that person will likely bring down the rest of the ship in the process.

Perhaps healthcare organizations hesitate to use RJPs because they don't want to hang out their dirty laundry. If they were taking the steps and measures discussed in this and the last chapter, however, they would have none to hang, and RJPs would just remind potential employees of stressors they already know about. Moreover, the use of RJPs might give an organization a chance to tout the many ways it is addressing those stressors. Just because it is a realistic preview doesn't mean it has to be all negative. It can describe the stressors and then follow up with steps that have been taken to address them. For example, the RJP could briefly explain the innovative scheduling systems the organization (or more accurately, its stress management team) has developed to deal with concerns over the interference of odd work schedules with family life. The RJP could even tout that the organization has a team dedicated to ensuring that stressors in the workplace are quickly addressed.

Mike Buckley of the University of Oklahoma has proposed an alternative approach to RJPs that may be similarly effective. His expectation-lowering procedures (ELPs) focus more generally on high expectations without delving into the details of the job (see Buckley et al. 1998). His approach includes simple statements asking job applicants to critically examine their expectations for the job before applying, reminding them that many people have unrealistically high expectations for jobs. In his studies, Buckley has found that these statements can be as effective as RJPs, with the advantage of being much shorter and usable for almost any job in the organization. ELPs may be a useful option for organizations seeking a quick, efficient route for management of expectations. That said, given that they will be analyzing the internal challenges and hopefully developing interventions to address them, organizations may want to develop full-fledged RJPs based on that analysis so that they can address the challenges with job applicants head-on.

PUTTING IT TOGETHER: STRESS-REDUCING HUMAN RESOURCES MANAGEMENT BUNDLES

Tony Wheeler (2008), a researcher at the University of Rhode Island, has taken the human resources management (HRM) techniques for reducing stress a step further and suggested that practices such as RJP and ELP can be implemented together, or *bundled*, to create stress-free work environments. He based this idea on the growing literature on high-performance work systems, suggesting that by considering the role of stress at multiple levels of an organization's structure, we can obtain high performance through lower stress. Specifically, he focused on HRM functions such as job analysis, proper RN staffing ratios, a multiple-hurdle selection system, formal socialization programs, performance management, job-based training, and progressive compensation systems. While his ideas were developed to apply primarily to nursing, most of them are relevant to all healthcare professions (including administrators).

Key Components of Stress-Reducing Human Resources Management Bundles
- Job analysis
- Proper RN staffing ratios
- Realistic job previews/expectation-lowering procedures
- Multiple-hurdle selection system
- Formal socialization programs
- Job-based training
- Development opportunities
- Performance management
- Progressive compensation systems

Wheeler's system begins with a proper job analysis, which is the foundation of any strong HRM system. Everything on the list in the preceding box is dependent on a clear understanding of the requirements of the job and a match between the knowledge, skills, and abilities (KSAs) of the employee and those requirements. As Wheeler (2008) notes, the persistent concerns with job design in healthcare suggest that care has not been taken to analyze the requirements of the job. For example, many unintended negative consequences of technology emerge because nobody has carefully determined what is required to use the technology and matched the KSAs of employees to those requirements.

As already discussed, proper RN staffing ratios have a key impact on stress and quality of care. The literature offers suggestions regarding the appropriate ratio of RNs to LPNs, as well as the proper ratio of RNs to patients (although this ratio varies according to patient acuity; see Kovner et al. [2002] and Person et al. [2004]).

Many organizations have addressed this problem by developing in-house flex pools that enable facilities to move personnel into areas that need the most staffing at a given moment. In addition to reducing stress through staff reinforcement, these pools personally benefit nurses who prefer a more flexible work schedule. Flex pools often offer options for working reduced hours or nontypical hours so nurses can maintain a balance between work and family life. Thus, such programs help full-time nurses by providing backup at key times and help flex pool nurses maintain a work–life balance.

A multiple-hurdle selection system involves the use of multiple tests to screen prospective employees. With each successive test, the selection of eligible candidates narrows. These tests should be based on the job analysis. Initial tests may involve basic qualifications for the job; later tests might focus more specifically on whether the applicant is a good fit for the job (e.g., Does the applicant's personality fit the type of patients he or she will be working with?). The interview should be among the last tests. Interviews refine the determination of fit even further and, thus, can help reduce future stress on the job (Wheeler et al. 2005).

Once someone has been hired, formal socialization programs are required to manage expectations (as discussed earlier) and integrate the employee into the organization's culture. The research literature suggests that socialization programs can be primary transmitters of employee culture, and programs that emphasize the organization's culture as well as networking opportunities among employees seem to improve the fit between the employee and his or her job more effectively than more passive forms of socialization (e.g., passing out an employee handbook or conducting a brief online training session). In turn, improved fit reduces stress (see Autry and Wheeler [2005] and Cable and Parsons [2001]). In other words, the organization's core values need to be clearly communicated to employees within their first year of working in the organization. These messages need to be delivered intentionally; they cannot be relayed "by accident" through passive forms of communication. Regular events should be held for new employees during their first year to help them adopt the values of the organization, including the development of a supportive environment.

One approach to cultural integration is to develop cohorts of new employees as they join the organization. Regardless of occupation or unit, they can be assigned to small groups (of about six to ten people) for informal meetings. Food is always a big draw for participation, so consider offering lunch. At these meetings, you can openly discuss the organization's values. As the groups mature, you can discuss the stressors they are encountering and how they are coping with them. This discussion can support your identification processes in the BRIDGES program. This approach does two things for employees: (1) It gives them clear information about the organization's values and an opportunity to explore how their own values align with them, and (2) it gives them an opportunity to network with others from across the organization.

In addition to involvement in the socialization program, employees need adequate training. Training is a delicate subject for many employees because they are reticent to admit that they don't have adequate KSAs to complete their jobs. Training programs, even when they are based on some sort of clinical or practicum experience, are unable to address all the contextual nuances of a job. Thus, while many healthcare professionals may be technically sound, they still struggle on the job because of aspects of the work or tasks specific to the workplace. Lack of training in these areas sets them up for failure and is a significant stressor. Think about your own position. Did you know everything about the job when you started? How long was your learning curve before you felt up to speed? (Perhaps you are still waiting for that day!) I have yet to talk with someone who was able to hit the ground running on the first day of his job; there are always things people could not know before starting.

How can we identify areas in which employees need training? A good job analysis can help you with this task, but discussion with employees about what they wish they knew when they started will help, too. Ask them to document the KSAs they needed but didn't have the first day on the job. These notes can be used to develop training programs or, at the very least, be passed along to new employees so they are aware that there are KSAs that they don't yet have but will need to develop at some point.

These thoughts lead to the next piece of the bundle—development opportunities. Most healthcare professionals are intimately familiar with the grind of fulfilling continuing education requirements and do so by way of the path of least resistance. Are we really developing skills, then, or are we just checking off a chore on our to-do list? Healthcare professionals crave true development, the kind that pushes them to think and broaden their horizons. In the same way that discussion with employees can pinpoint training opportunities, discussion with healthcare professionals can elicit development opportunities. Even more gratifying for employees is to have them create new development programs for others. Employees feel empowered when they are asked to develop the skills of other employees. This form of development is particularly enriching in that the ultimate learner in the process is the one doing the teaching.

Contrary to popular belief, annual performance appraisals are not effective in managing employee performance. They are a significant source of stress for all involved. Furthermore, they are so sanitized so as not to hurt anyone's feelings that they no longer serve their original purpose (to provide meaningful feedback to employees) or their debased purpose (to document bad behavior in case someone needs to be fired). As a result, they have become almost worthless.

Rather than scheduling that awkward annual meeting, document and give regular feedback that reinforces positive behaviors. Problematic behavior should be documented as well, but keep in mind that, according to learning theory and research, people react better to positive reinforcement. Punishment tends to prompt avoidant behaviors, not change for the better. When emphasis is placed on what employees do wrong, they don't know what they need to do to improve. Saying "you filled that prescription incorrectly" doesn't tell people how to fill it correctly and offers little information on how to change their behavior.

The focus on negative behavior in performance appraisals and the avoidant behavior that results partly account for why medical errors have become such a problem. If you knew that an error was going to appear on your next appraisal, would you report it? You might, in part because if you didn't, you could jeopardize your position, your license, and so forth. What about near misses? Information on near misses is extremely valuable but rarely reported. Exemplary organizations make a concerted effort to reward employees for reporting near misses and treat these instances as opportunities to solve a problem before it becomes a bigger problem. Such positive feedback guides people in the right direction.

An outgrowth of performance management is progressive compensation systems. Compensation reflects what the organization values and rewards the behavior it wants repeated. Accordingly, it is a source of stress for employees. Healthcare professionals who work long or nonstandard hours and require a great deal of training and skill often feel undercompensated. One solution may be to simply pay higher wages. Mark Brown, a researcher at Bradley University, found that hospitals with leading pay policies (meaning they pay above-average wages) had higher performance, likely because they are able to attract better talent (see Brown, Sturman, and Simmering [2003] and Brown [2006]). The problem, however, is that as more hospitals fight for talent, the bar is raised, and having a leading policy becomes not only more expensive but expected (Upenieks 2005).

Thus, to sustain effective performance management, organizations need to consider more progressive forms of compensation. Interestingly, some forms of compensation not only reward excellent performance but also can address workplace stressors. For example, a significant stressor among healthcare professionals, in part because of nonstandard working hours, is work–family conflict (Duffield, Pallas, and Aiken 2004). Health professionals often feel that their time at work is detracting from time that could be spent with family. Moreover, the strains of work can carry over to home life; some may actually take out some of their frustrations from work on their family.

Benefits that help balance work and family life can play a significant role in attracting top-quality professionals and reducing their stress. Compressed workweeks have been one solution for many healthcare professionals. Although they make for somewhat longer working days, they allow for longer stretches with family (Havlovic, Lau, and Pinfield 2002). Other benefits such as child care, elder care, and employee assistance programs also help employees balance work and family life and may offer a slight advantage in attracting healthcare professionals.

The point of this discussion is to explain the necessity of constructing an HR profile—a bundle—that not only includes many of the best HRM practices from the literature but also provides an edge in preventing stress. These bundles will help your BRIDGES program develop longer-term sustainability.

TAKEAWAY POINTS: DEVELOPING A "STRESS-FREE ENVIRONMENT"

Unfortunately, implementation of the BRIDGES program described in Chapter 5 is not enough to deal with stress long term. To sustain a positive environment and keep it stress free (or at least stress reduced), you will need to use some of the techniques outlined in this chapter. Because healthcare organizations traditionally have regarded the HR department not as playing a strategic role but fulfilling more of an administrative role, a focus on HR strategies may seem odd. Changing this perception will have a significant positive impact on stress. The idea of HR as a department must be replaced by the idea of HR as an asset. No healthcare facility in the world can function without the KSAs of humans, yet we do so little to develop them. Use of the techniques suggested in this chapter will foster KSAs in a way that will also reduce stress over the long term.

Here are three main points to take away from this chapter:

- Lack of support is a major source of stress and burnout in healthcare. Development of a supportive culture will help address this problem over the long term.
- Unmet expectations are also a major stressor. Simple techniques, such as the use of RJPs and ELPs, can help reduce this problem.
- Bundles of the best-known HR practices that can help reduce stress include
  - job analysis,
  - proper RN staffing ratios,
  - RJPs/ELPs,
  - the multiple-hurdle selection system,
  - formal socialization programs,
  - job-based training,
  - development opportunities,
  - performance management, and
  - progressive compensation systems.

The final chapter will wrap things up by discussing how burned-out "workers" can become engaged professionals, and will set your organization forth on a positive path toward a stress-free future.

CHAPTER 7

Putting It All Together: Beating Burnout, Building Engagement

When I wake up in the morning, the first thing I think about is work. That used to be a bad thing. It used to make me want to roll back over and hit snooze. But now I'm excited to get started, excited to see what my day will bring.

—Pharmacist working in an academic medical center

I like that when I go to work, I look up at the clock and don't realize that the day has passed me by.

—Urologist working in a community hospital

YOU HAVE REACHED a critical point in your journey toward a healthier workplace. You have evaluated a difficult work environment, turned it around, and established long-term structures to sustain employee well-being. You could stop there. You have eliminated, or at least reduced, your employees' burnout, and they no longer mind going to work. However, by stopping at this point, you might limit their potential, and although they don't mind going to work, their work remains unfulfilling.

On the other hand, you can continue. You can develop an engaged workforce—a group of employees who thrive at work, who are excited about work because they feel it is their calling, not just something they do to make a living.

THE WELL-BEING CONTINUUM: GOING FROM "NOT BURNED OUT" TO "ENGAGED" IN WORK

The term *engagement* is kicked around a lot, especially in healthcare, partly as a result of recent efforts by influential bodies (such as the Malcolm Baldrige National Quality Program) to recognize workforce issues. Unfortunately, this term has not been clearly defined, so it means different things to different people. For example, the Baldrige Criteria define engagement in terms of commitment to the organization's goals and mission. Researchers have studied engagement for many years, defining it simply as "commitment." Whether commitment is really engagement, however, is debatable. For example, as a professor, I am committed to universities' goal to educate citizens. I think it is a critical mission, but that doesn't mean I have been engaged in every job I've had.

Engagement is more than just commitment to the organization's mission. Wilmar Schaufeli and colleagues (2002) define engagement in terms of three qualities:

- *Vigor*—the energy that one brings to the job. Engaged individuals bring a lot of energy to their work.
- *Dedication*—the commitment aspect of engagement. Dedicated employees are interested in advancing the organization's mission.
- *Absorption*—a state in which an individual is engrossed in work. Absorption is sometimes called *flow* and is often manifested as losing track of time as a result of being fully immersed in a task.

Organizations want employees to be engaged. Research suggests that engaged employees perform at higher levels and are less likely to leave the organization. As the first quote opening the chapter suggests, engaged employees wake up in the morning and *want* to go to work. Healthcare organizations want to employ these kinds of people, not only because they will be highly productive but because they will truly satisfy the patients with whom they interact. They will take time to ensure the patient is receiving the highest quality of care possible. They will be sure to follow patient safety procedures because they recognize their importance.

How does engagement lead to all of these behaviors? It does so as a result of having a lot of extra resources. People are engaged when they have sufficient time and motivation to do their work right; when they have the support of their supervisors, colleagues, and family; and when they have the KSAs needed to get the job done. Per the conservation of resources theory, if people have excess resources, they have more resources to invest. As they invest those resources in positive ways, their investments pay off in even more positive ways, creating a virtuous cycle of resource gains.

This discussion has shown the importance of taking that next step. You don't want to stop at the point where you've reduced burnout; you want to push ahead so that you can develop a highly engaged workforce. You want to take the next step because it is in the best interest of your employees, your patients, and yourself.

ADDRESSING BURNOUT BUILDS ENGAGEMENT

The title of this section does not mean that by addressing burnout you have developed engagement. Burnout and engagement are related, parallel processes, not two ends of the same continuum. A point can be reached at which burnout has been eliminated, but elimination of burnout does not automatically transform into engagement. At the point where burnout no longer exists, you will need to switch over to a parallel, positive process of developing engagement (see Exhibit 7.1).

Exhibit 7.1 Burnout and Engagement as Parallel Processes

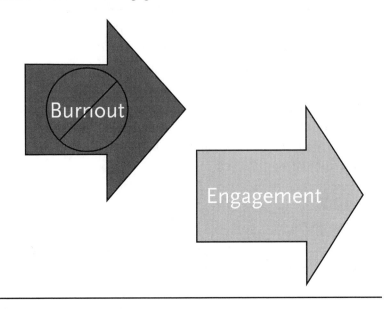

The process involved in developing engagement is similar to that involved in addressing burnout. Because engagement results from excess resources and burnout results from a lack of resources (or a threat to our resources, such as word of layoffs or a bad investment of resources), the solution to both is to enhance employees' resources.

However, a little more work is required to develop engagement than that required to reduce stress. While many of the resources that help reduce stress will also help develop engagement, the latter is more challenging in that you may need to broaden the resources. You can use this task to your advantage in a variety of ways. For example, you have already created a team to address stressors in the workplace. Engaged employees will want to participate in more of these types of activities. While you can reach a point where you create so many committees that they overlap and people begin to question their value, engaged employees will want the opportunity to participate.

To foster this type of engagement, you will need to give up a significant amount of the control associated with your management title. Allowing employees to self-manage and self-organize will lead to a more engaged workforce and better overall outcomes. This progression is consistent with the emerging science of complex adaptive systems, which has now been appropriately applied to healthcare. Self-organization of systems fosters engagement, while engagement fosters further positive self-organization, creating a virtuous resource cycle like the one described earlier.

In addition to giving up control, you'll need to provide the same resource that was so important in dealing with burnout: social support. For employees to feel that they are capable of self-organization, they need plenty of emotional and instrumental support. They need to know that their decisions will be supported and that resources will be available to support the reasonable decisions they make. They need to be rewarded to reinforce the supportive behaviors they show to each other.

At first glance, this initiative seems expensive. However, most employees are sensitive to the financial implications of their decisions. They keep personal budgets. They know that execution of a decision involves costs. Further, by improving the work process, they will save you money over the long run. They will make the organization safer, reduce turnover, and increase patient satisfaction. These outcomes will save you more money than you realize. Moreover, engaged employees will help you reduce management costs. You will be able to spend less time organizing and controlling and more time on other endeavors, such as marketing and development.

If you have implemented the other structures discussed in the book, you are in a good position to continue to develop your workforce into one that is highly engaged. You will be glad you took the initiative to the next level.

FINAL TAKEAWAY POINTS: BUILDING BRIDGES

We have reached the end of our discussion—but not our work. To review, this book was based on three principles:

- Everyone experiences stress, but not everyone experiences burnout.
- While everyone has a unique reaction to stress, people tend to experience the same stressors.
- People know what is causing their stress, and they likely know the solution, too.

To address these three principles, I proposed the BRIDGES framework, which involves healthcare professionals in addressing their burnout. Full implementation of this program will take significant time and resources, but remember that thousands, if not millions, of dollars are lost annually as a result of the negative effects of stress and burnout.

You have nothing to lose. You have only to gain a productive, safe organization with engaged employees who stay with you for the long haul—a challenging goal, but one worth pursuing.

Appendix A

Helpful Resources for Dealing with Stress and Burnout

THE FOLLOWING RESOURCES supplement this text and provide relevant, interesting information about work-related stress and burnout.

WEBSITES

A variety of organizations have developed websites about work stress and burnout. Some are more work-specific and research-focused than others.

The American Psychological Association (APA) website includes a topics page about stress. Its content is general (e.g., it includes information about stress between couples in a relationship), but it provides many useful reports and media links to stories about stress. It can be accessed at www.apa.org/topics/topicstress.html.

The National Institute for Occupational Safety and Health (NIOSH) has become interested in the topic of stress as an occupational health concern. As such, it has set up a site with stress resources, including its report, *Stress...At Work* (www.cdc.gov/niosh/docs/99-101). From this website, you can order additional stress resources, including a short video about stress. The main site can be accessed at www.cdc.gov/niosh/topics/stress. The NIOSH website also includes resources about work schedules and their impact on stress and health. (For example, you may recall a study conducted a few years back about the impact that extended schedules have on interns' risk of involvement in car crashes.) Given the significant impact that scheduling can have on healthcare professionals, you may find these resources useful. They can be accessed at www.cdc.gov/niosh/topics/workschedules. Last, the NIOSH website includes tools for measuring quality of work life (see www.cdc.gov/niosh/topics/stress/qwlquest.html). You may find this measure useful as you identify challenges in the workplace.

The American Institute of Stress was established over 30 years ago to provide resources about stress. The Institute's reports on stress can be accessed through its website (www.stress.org), and members can access additional resources, such as monthly newsletters.

BOOKS AND OTHER READINGS

Books Outlining Theories Discussed in This Book

The following books outline Hobfoll's conservation of resources theory. They detail the reasoning and evidence behind his theory, including his work in trauma research:

Hobfoll, S. E. 2001. "The Influence of Culture, Community, and the Nested Self in the Stress Process: Advancing Conservation of Resources Theory." *Applied Psychology: An International Review* 50: 337–70.
———. 1998. *Stress, Culture, and Community*. New York: Plenum.
———. 1988. *The Ecology of Stress*. New York: Hemisphere.

The following books provide greater detail on the transaction model of stress and coping:

Lazarus, R. S. 1966. *Psychological Stress and the Coping Process.* New York: McGraw-Hill.

Lazarus, R. S., and S. Folkman. 1984. *Stress, Appraisal, and Coping.* New York: Springer.

Books Outlining Action Research Approaches

Although each book takes a slightly different approach to action research (e.g., they include different steps), they all follow the same basic principles of integrating employees in the process:

Bartunek, J., T. Costa, R. Dame, and D. LeLacheur. 2000. "Managers and Project Leaders Conducting Their Own Action Research Interventions." In *Handbook of Organizational Consultation,* 2nd edition, edited by R. T. Golembiewski, 59–70. New York: Marcel Dekker.

Bruce, R., and S. Wyman. 1998. *Changing Organizations: Practicing Action Training and Research.* Thousand Oaks, CA: Sage.

McNiff, J. 2002. *Action Research: Principles and Practice.* London: Routledge.

———. 2000. *Action Research in Organizations.* London: Routledge.

Reason, P., and H. Bradbury. 2001. *The Handbook of Action Research.* London: Sage.

Stringer, E. T. 1999. *Action Research,* 2nd edition. Thousand Oaks, CA: Sage.

Other Excellent Stress-Related Books

Cooper, C. L., and P. Dewe. 2004. *Stress: A Brief History.* Oxford: Blackwell. (An excellent historical treatment of the study of

stress; research focused, but provides a nice overview of the
literature as it developed)

Halbesleben, J. R. B. 2008. *Handbook of Stress and Burnout in
Health Care*. New York: Nova Science. (An edited academic
volume focusing on the academic study of stress and burnout
within the healthcare industry; features chapters by some of
the world's top researchers on the topic)

Leiter, M. P., and C. Maslach. 2005. *Banishing Burnout: Six
Strategies for Improving Your Relationship with Work*. San
Francisco: Jossey-Bass. (A presentation by Leiter and Maslach,
pioneers in the study of burnout, of an alternative, more self-
help approach that encourages individuals to deal with the
burnout-inducing environments in which they work; differs
from the BRIDGES program in that BRIDGES focuses on
changing the environment to avoid burnout in the first place)

Schaufeli, W., and D. Enzmann. 1998. *The Burnout Companion
to Study and Practice*. London: Taylor and Francis. (While
now a bit dated, an excellent overview of the burnout literature; not necessarily focused on healthcare organizations,
though much of the literature applies)

Wainwright, D., and M. Calnan. 2002. *Work Stress: The Making
of a Modern Epidemic*. New York: Open University Press. (An
exploration of the sociological perspective of stress, based on
the authors' qualitative research on stress, emotions, and
health; a fascinating glimpse into the changing perspectives
on stress over time and the advent of the "work stress victim")

OTHER RESOURCE OPPORTUNITIES

Conferences and workshops are available that focus on state-of-the-art
mechanisms for reducing stress. Now that you have some background
on evidence-based approaches to stress and burnout, particularly
with regard to intervention, carefully consider the perspective of
the workshop and the presenter. Many of these workshops are not

based on sound theory or science and are of little use in the long run.

That said, some good options exist. Every other year, APA and NIOSH co-host a conference on work stress and health. You can find more information on past and future conferences at www.apa.org/pi/work/wsh.html. In addition to presentations by academics conducting stress research, there are workshops on stress intervention techniques, "ask an expert" sessions in which you might procure advice specific to your organization, and other sessions you might find useful. It may even be a great place to present an evaluation of your own stress reduction/prevention program based on this book. Plus, you can meet me there!

Appendix B

BRIDGES Resources

THE FOLLOWING FORMS are provided to help you organize your BRIDGES processes.

BUILDING RELATIONSHIPS FORM

The form in Exhibit B.1 is designed for the relationship-building stage. It will help you (1) track the people you talk with and the areas you visit and (2) begin collecting data on existing and potential challenges.

Exhibit B.1 Building Relationships Form

Unit/department visited: _____Date: _____Time: _____
Whom you talked with: _____
Observations during visit (e.g., potential challenges):

Integration: How does this visit fit with others you have completed? Are any themes emerging?

INTERVIEW FORM

The form in Exhibit B.2 is only a starting point. It should be tailored to suit the needs of your organization.

Exhibit B.2

As you may be aware, we have created a task force dedicated to addressing stress and burnout at our facility. We are using interviews to collect information about stress from employees so we can work together to develop solutions to these issues.

1. What are the primary challenges you face in doing your job?
2. How often do you face those challenges?
3. What suggestions do you have for addressing those challenges?
4. Clarify your suggestions.
5. How would we implement them?
6. Who would be responsible for implementing them?
7. What resources would we need to implement them?
8. What do you enjoy about your job?
9. Aside from the suggestions you made in question #3, what could make your job even better?

Thank you for your candid feedback. If you have any further suggestions for our task force, please contact me at _____.

SEVEN TIPS FOR RUNNING SUCCESSFUL STRESS FOCUS GROUPS

1. Select a group that will maximize outcomes.
    a. Too large a group will lead to diminishing returns. Do not select more than 12 people.

b. Choose people who will remain positive and provide meaningful solutions. Devil's advocates might be valuable but will need to be managed so that they do not short circuit the group.

2. Establish rapport quickly. Introduce yourself and have the group use name tags.

3. Establish ground rules.

   a. Explain the purpose of the group (e.g., "We're seeking solutions, not just griping.").

   b. Level the playing field. (No one's ideas are necessarily better than anyone else's.)

4. Record the session.

   a. For this type of project, exact recordings are usually not necessary.

   b. Work in pairs; appoint one moderator and one note taker.

5. Focus on idea development.

   a. Probe for more information if participants propose vague ideas.

   b. If the group is reluctant to talk, use an idea heard earlier (e.g., in earlier focus groups) to generate discussion. You may also want to develop a few ideas of your own to offer for feedback if the group does not have ideas to bring to the table.

6. Facilitate more than participate.

   a. Limit your own participation.

   b. Don't encourage one idea over another.

7. Wrap up the session and communicate next steps.

   a. Summarize the discussion.

   b. Clarify any confusion you have about the participants' suggestions.

   c. Explain the remainder of the BRIDGES program and how the task force will proceed.

References

American Psychological Association. 2007. "Stress in America." [Online report; retrieved 7/7/09.] http://apahelpcenter.media room.com/file.php/138/Stress+in+America+REPORT+FINAL .doc.

American Institute of Stress. 2009. "Stress in the Workplace, Job Stress, Occupational Stress, Job Stress Questionnaire." [Online information; retrieved 9/15/09.] www.stress.org/ topic-workplace.htm.

Autry, C. A., and A. R. Wheeler. 2005. "Post-Hire Human Resource Management Practices and Person-Organization Fit: A Study of Blue-Collar Employees." *Journal of Managerial Issues* 17 (1): 58–75.

Bakker, A. B., W. B. Schaufeli, H. J. Sixma, W. Bosveld, and D. van Dierendonck. 2000. "Patient Demands, Lack of Reciprocity, and Burnout: A Five-Year Longitudinal Study Among General Practitioners." *Journal of Organizational Behavior* 21 (4): 425–41.

Boffa, D. P., and P. Pawola. 2006. "Identification and Conceptualization of Nurse Super Users." *Journal of Healthcare Information Management* 20 (4): 60–68.

Brown, M. P. 2006. "The Effect of Nursing Professional Pay Structures and Pay Levels on Hospitals' Heart Attack Outcomes." *Health Care Management Review* 31 (3): 1–10.

Brown, M. P., M. C. Sturman, and M. J. Simmering. 2003. "Compensation Policy and Organizational Performance: The Efficiency, Operational, and Financial Implications of Pay Levels and Pay Structure." *Academy of Management Journal* 46 (6): 752–62.

Bruce, R., and S. Wyman. 1998. *Changing Organizations: Practicing Action Training and Research.* Thousand Oaks, CA: Sage.

Buckley, M. R., D. B. Fedor, J. G. Veres, D. S. Wiese, and S. M. Carraher. 1998. "Investigating Newcomer Expectations and Job-Related Outcomes." *Journal of Applied Psychology* 83 (3): 452–61.

Cable, D. M., and C. K. Parsons. 2001. "Socialization Tactics and Person–Organization Fit." *Personnel Psychology* 54 (1): 1–23.

Cheng, Y., I. Kowachi, E. H. Coakley, J. Schwartz, and G. Colditz. 2000. "Association Between Psychosocial Work Characteristics and Health Functioning in American Women: Prospective Study." *British Medical Journal* 320 (7247): 1432–36.

Cohen, S., T. Kamarck, and R. Mermelstein. 1983. "A Global Measure of Perceived Stress." *Journal of Health and Social Behavior* 24 (4): 385–96.

Demerouti, E., A. B. Bakker, I. Vardakou, and A. Kantas. 2002. "The Convergent Validity of Two Burnout Instruments: A Multitrait-Multimethod Analysis." *European Journal of Psychological Assessment* 18: 296–307.

Duffield, C., L. O. Pallas, and L. M. Aiken. 2004. "Nurses Who Work Outside Nursing." *Journal of Advanced Nursing* 47 (6): 664–71.

Fillion, L., and L. Saint-Laurent. 2003. "Stressors Linked to Palliative Care Nursing: The Importance of Organizational, Professional, and Emotional Support." [Online report; retrieved 7/10/09.] www.chsrf.ca/final_research/ogc/fillion _e.php.

French, S. E., R. Lenton, V. Walters, and J. Eyles. 2000. "An Empirical Evaluation of the Expanded Nursing Stress Scale." *Journal of Nursing Measurement* 8 (2): 161–78.

Gray-Toft, P., and J. G. Anderson. 1981. "The Nursing Stress Scale: Development of an Instrument." *Journal of Behavioral Assessment* 3 (1): 11–23.

Halbesleben, J. R. B. 2006a. "Patient Reciprocity and Physician Burnout: What Do Patients Bring to the Patient–Physician Relationship?" *Health Services Management Research* 19 (4): 215–22.

———. 2006b. "Sources of Social Support and Burnout: A Meta-Analytic Test of the Conservation of Resources Model." *Journal of Applied Psychology* 91 (5): 1134–45.

Halbesleben, J. R. B., H. K. Osburn, and M. D. Mumford. 2006. "Action Research as a Burnout Intervention: Reducing Burnout in the Federal Fire Service." *Journal of Applied Behavioral Science* 42 (2): 244–66.

Halbesleben, J. R. B., and C. Rathert. 2008. "Linking Physician Burnout and Patient Outcomes: Exploring the Dyadic Relationship Between Physicians and Patients." *Health Care Management Review* 33 (1): 29–39.

Halbesleben, J. R. B., B. J. Wakefield, D. S. Wakefield, and L. Cooper. 2008. "Nurse Burnout and Patient Safety Outcomes: Nurse Safety Perception vs. Reporting Behavior." *Western Journal of Nursing Research* 30 (5): 560–77.

Halbesleben, J. R. B., D. S. Wakefield, M. M. Ward, J. Brokel, and D. Crandall. 2009. "The Relationship Between Super Users' Attitudes and Employee Experiences with Clinical Information Systems." *Medical Care Research and Review* 66 (1): 82–96.

Havlovic, S. J., D. C. Lau, and L. T. Pinfield. 2002. "Repercussions of Work Schedule Congruence Among Full-Time, Part-Time, and Contingent Nurses." *Health Care Management Review* 27 (4): 30–41.

Hobfoll, S. E. 1988. *The Ecology of Stress.* New York: Hemisphere.

Holmes, T. H., and R. H. Rahe. 1967. "The Social Readjustment Rating Scale." *Journal of Psychosomatic Research* 11 (2): 213–18.

Jones, C. B. 2008. "Revisiting Nurse Turnover Costs: Adjusting for Inflation." *Journal of Nursing Administration* 38 (1): 11–18.

Jones, J. W. 1980. *Preliminary Manual: The Staff Burnout Scale for Health Professionals.* Park Ridge, IL: London House.

Kovner, C., C. Jones, C. Zhan, P. J. Gergen, and J. Basu. 2002. "Nurse Staffing and Postsurgical Adverse Events: An Analysis of Administrative Data from a Sample of U.S. Hospitals, 1990–1996." *Health Services Research* 37 (3): 611–29.

Kristensen, T. S., M. Borritz, E. Villadsen, and K. B. Christensen. 2005. "The Copenhagen Burnout Inventory: A New Tool for the Assessment of Burnout." *Work and Stress* 19 (3): 192–207.

Lazarus, R. S., and S. Folkman. 1984. *Stress, Appraisal, and Coping.* New York: Springer.

LePine, J. A., N. P. Podsakoff, and M. A. LePine. 2005. "A Meta-Analytic Test of the Challenge Stressor-Hindrance Stressor Framework: An Explanation for Inconsistent Relationships Among Stressors and Performance." *Academy of Management Journal* 48 (5): 764–75.

Maslach, C. 1982. *Burnout: The Cost of Caring.* Englewood Cliffs, NJ: Prentice Hall.

Maslach, C., and S. Jackson. 1981. "The Measurement of Experienced Burnout." *Journal of Occupational Behavior* 2: 99–113.

McVicar, A. 2003. "Workplace Stress in Nursing: A Literature Review." *Journal of Advanced Nursing* 44 (6): 633–42.

Melamed, S., A. Shirom, S. Toker, S. Berliner, and L. Shapira. 2006. "Burnout and Risk of Cardiovascular Disease: Evidence, Possible Causal Paths, and Promising Research Directions." *Psychological Bulletin* 132 (3): 327–53.

Mercer, M., T. Szaniawski, and J. Guettler. 2002. "Slashing Turnover Costs." [Online article; retrieved 7/8/09.] www.hrgrouponline.com/article2.html.

National Institute for Occupational Safety and Health (NIOSH). 1999. "Stress at Work." [Online publication; retrieved 7/7/09.] www.cdc.gov/niosh/docs/99-101.

Neveu, J.-P. 2008. "Burnout and Consequences: A Review of Health Professional Maltreatment to the Patient." In *Handbook of Stress and Burnout in Health Care*, edited by J. R. B. Halbesleben. New York: Nova Science Publishers.

Person, S. D., J. J. Allison, C. I. Kiefe, M. T. Weaver, O. D. Williams, R. M. Centor, and N. W. Weissman. 2004. "Nurse Staffing and Mortality for Medicare Patients with Acute Myocardial Infarction." *Medical Care* 42 (1): 4–12.

PricewaterhouseCoopers. 2007. "What Works: Healing the Healthcare Staffing Shortage." [Online report; retrieved 2/23/09.] www.pwc.com/extweb/pwcpublications.nsf/docid/674D1E79A678A0428525730D006B74A9.

Sabongui, A. G. 2006. "Stress and Burnout." [Online article; retrieved 7/9/09.] www.wellnessprosalliance.com/pdfs/Stress_and_Burnout.pdf.

Schaufeli, W. B., M. P. Leiter, C. Maslach, and S. E. Jackson. 1996. "The Maslach Burnout Inventory—General Survey." In *Maslach Burnout Inventory*, edited by C. Maslach, S. E. Jackson, and M. P. Leiter. Palo Alto, CA: Consulting Psychologists Press.

Schaufeli, W. B., M. Salanova, V. González-Romá, and A. B. Bakker. 2002. "The Measurement of Engagement and Burnout: A Confirmative Analytic Approach." *Journal of Happiness Studies* 3: 71–92.

Schloss, E. P., D. M. Flanagan, C. L. Culler, and A. L. Wright. 2009. "Some Hidden Costs of Faculty Turnover in Clinical Departments in One Academic Medical Center." *Academic Medicine* 84 (1): 32–36.

Shirom, A., and S. Melamed. 2006. "A Comparison of the Construct Validity of Two Burnout Measures in Two Groups of Professionals." *International Journal of Stress Management* 13 (2): 176–200.

Stoller, J. K., D. K. Orens, and L. Kester. 2001. "The Impact of Turnover Among Respiratory Care Practitioners in a Health Care System: Frequency and Associated Costs." *Respiratory Care* 46 (3): 238–42.

Stordeur, S., W. D'Hoore, and C. Vandenberghe. 2001. "Leadership, Organizational Stress, and Emotional Exhaustion Among Hospital Nursing Staff." *Journal of Advanced Nursing* 35 (4): 533–42.

Studer, Q. 2004. *Hardwiring Excellence: Purpose, Worthwhile Work, Making a Difference.* Gulf Breeze, FL: Fire Starter Publishing.

Upenieks, V. 2005. "Recruitment and Retention Strategies: A Magnet Hospital Prevention Model." *Nursing Economic$* 21 (1): 7–13.

Van Dierendonck, D., W. B. Schaufeli, and B. P. Buunk. 1998. "The Evaluation of an Individual Burnout Intervention Program: The Role of Inequity and Social Support." *Journal of Applied Psychology* 83 (3): 392–407.

Wainwright, D., and M. Calnan. 2002. *Work Stress: The Making of a Modern Epidemic.* Buckingham, UK: Open University Press.

Wheeler, A. R. 2008. "Disconnecting the Stress-Burnout-Turnover Relationship Among Nursing Professionals: A Synthesis of Micro and Macro HRM Research." In *Handbook of Stress and Burnout in Health Care*, edited by J. R. B. Halbesleben, 187–99. New York: Nova Science Publishers.

Wheeler, A. R., M. R. Buckley, J. R. Halbesleben, R. L. Brouer, and G. R. Ferris. 2005. "'The Elusive Criterion of Fit' Revisited: Toward an Integrative Theory of MDF." In *Research in Personnel and Human Resource Management*, vol. 24, edited by J. Martocchio, 265–304. Greenwich, CT: Elsevier/JAI Press.

Index

Absorption, in work, 96

Abuse, of patients, 14

Action research, definition of, 58

Action research programs: for burnout reduction, 57; action/reflection cycle component of, 59–60, 69; participants deeply embedded in, 58–59

Administrative staff, stressors among, 27–29

Administrators, stress experienced by, xi–xii

Age factors, in burnout, 39–40

American Institute of Stress, 8

American Psychological Association, 6–7

Appraisal, of stressful situations, 18–20, 31

Arousal, 1–2

Assessment: of burnout, 40, 43, 46–50, 51; of stress, 43–46, 51, 97–99

Attention deficit hyperactivity disorder (ADHD), 37

Autonomy, 41

Avoidant strategies, for coping with stress, 19, 29–30, 41

Baldrige National Quality Program, 96

Biofeedback, 45

Bradley University, 91

BRIDGES program: for burnout reduction, 60–77, 99–200; build relationships step, 60, 61, 62–66; design interventions step, 60, 61, 72–75; evaluate interventions step, 60, 61, 73–74; goal of, 61; identify step, 60, 61, 66–72, 89; implement interventions step, 60, 61, 75; resources for, 107–109; sustain change step, 60, 61, 75–76; time frame for, 72

Brown, Mark, 91

Buckley, Mike, 86

Burnout, 33–42; assessment of, 40, 43, 46–50, 51, 97–99; as continuum, 36; definition of, xviii, 31; disengagement component of, 33, 34–35, 41, 48; exhaustion component of, 33, 34–35, 41; experience of, 33–35; gender factors in,

39, 40; health consequences of, 5–6; as job dissatisfaction cause, 5; as job turnover cause, 5, 6; as lack of motivation cause, 3; negative impact on job performance, 2–3; organizational factors in, 38–40, 41; personal factors in, 36, 37–39, 41; prevention of, 79–80; protective factors against, 37–38; relationship to engagement, 97–99; social exchange model of, 38–93; stability of, 40–41; vicious cycle of, 7

Burnout intervention programs, 57; failure of, 72; individualized, 54–55, 56, 76; supportive work environment-based, 80–84

Burnout scores, variability in, 40

Canada, burnout-related disability claims in, 11

Canadian Health Services Research Foundation, 24

Cardiovascular disorders, stress-related, 6, 7, 37

Challenges, identification of, 68–71

Change, differentiated from improvement, 73, 74

Chief executive officers (CEOs), involvement in burnout reduction programs, 67

Clinical function, coordination of, 27–28

Clinical staff, stressors among, 23–27, 31

Colleagues, as social support, 37–38, 80–84

Commitment: differentiated from engagement, 95; effect of realistic job previews on, 85; lack of, xvi

Communication, among healthcare professionals, 25–26

Compensation, progressive, 91–92

Computerized physician order entry (CPOE), 73–74

Conflict: with colleagues, 25–26, 31; work–family, 91–92

Conservation of resources theory, of stress, 20–22, 31, 97

Consideration, individualized, 63

Consultants, employees' relationships with, 62–63

Continuing education, 90

Copenhagen Burnout Inventory, 49

Coping: with stress, xvii–xviii, 29-30; active, 19, 29, 30; avoidant, 19, 29–30, 41

Costs, stress-related, 8–9, 11–12

Crew resource management training, 29; evaluation of, 74

Crossing the Quality Chasm (Institute of Medicine), 60–61

Cultural integration, of new employees, 88–89

Cynicism, 34, 47

Data collection, in burnout reduction programs, 69–71

Dedication, 96

Deep breathing techniques, 56

Demerouti, Eva, 48

Depersonalization, 34, 47

Development programs, 90

Diabetes mellitus, burnout as risk factor for, 6, 7

Disability claims, 11–12

Disengagement, 33, 34–35, 41, 48

Dissatisfaction, differentiated from stress, xv–xvi

Eating habits, effect of stress on, 6–7

Efficacy, reduced personal, 35, 41, 47

Emotional stress, patient care-related, 24–25

Engagement: of the workforce, 95–99; differentiated from commitment, 95; qualities of, 96;

relationship to burnout, 97–99
Errors, medical: accountability for, 28; effect of performance appraisals on, 91; reporting of, 13–14, 28, 91
Evaluation: of burnout reduction interventions, 60, 61, 73–74; "happy-sheet" approach in, 74
Exhaustion, 33, 34–35, 41, 47, 48; as burnout intervention target, 55
Expectation-lowering procedures (ELPs), 86
Expectations: management of, 84–86; misaligned or unmet, 57, 84
Extraversion, 37

Family–work conflict, 91–92
Feedback, employees' access to, 38, 41
Fight-or-flight response, 19, 34–35
Firefighters, 58, 62, 68
Flex pools, 88
Focus groups, 70, 71–72, 108–109
Folkman, Susan, 18–20

Gender factors, in burnout, 39, 40

Hardiness, 37
Hardwiring for Excellence (Studer), 75
Harvard University, 5
Health, adverse effects of burnout on, 5–6
Healthcare, patients' participation in, 38–39
Healthcare costs, stress/burnout-related, 11–12, 14, 15
Healthcare professionals: conflict among, 25–26; consequences of stress among, 2–7; stress experienced by, xii
Healthcare professions, turnover-related costs in, 9
Health (magazine), xii
Hobfoll, Stevan, 20

Human resources departments, 67–68
Human resources management bundles, stress-reducing, 86–92
Hypotheses: regarding stress, 17–31; conservation of resources theory, 20–22, 31, 97; transaction stress model, 18–20, 31

Ideas, for burnout reduction, 65, 66
Identification: as burnout reduction program component, 60, 61, 66–72, 89; of challenges, 60, 61, 68–71; of opportunities, 60, 61, 71–72; of team members, 60, 61, 66–68
Improvement, differentiated from change, 73, 74
Incompetence, differentiated from stress, xvi–xvii
Individualized approaches, in burnout intervention, 54–55, 56
Infertility, burnout as risk factor for, 6
Information resources, for stress and burnout management, 101–105
Injuries: occupational, 4, 7; workers' compensation claims for, 12
Institute of Medicine (IOM), 28; *Crossing the Quality Chasm*, 60–61
Interviewing/interviews: in burnout reduction programs, 64–65, 71; stress, 11

Jackson, Susan, 47
Job analysis, 86–87, 89–90
Job applicants: expectation-lowering procedures (ELPs) for, 86; multiple-bundle selection system for, 88; realistic job previews (RJPs) for, 84, 86
Job dissatisfaction, burnout-related, 5

Kerr, Steven, 82–83

Knowledge, skills, and abilities
(KSAs), of employees, 87, 89,
90, 93, 97
Kristensen, T. S., 49

Lazarus, Richard, 18–20
Leadership: as stress source, 26, 27;
transactional, 26
Life events, as stressors, 44

Malcolm Baldrige National Quality
Program, 96
Management, by exception, 26
Managers: frontline, selection criteria
for, 26; role in stress management,
xix; stress experienced by, xi–xii
Marital status, effect on burnout risk,
37–38
Maslach, Christina, 33, 35, 47
Maslach Burnout Inventory (MBI),
47–48, 49
Medical departments, turnover-
related costs in, 9
Medical interns, stress experienced
by, xii
Meditation, 56
Meta-analysis, 80–81
Motivation, burnout-related decrease
in, 3
Motivational resources, 20–22, 31
Multiple-bundle selection system, 88

National Institute for Occupational
Safety and Health (NIOSH), 7;
Stress at Work report, xiv–xv, xvi,
36
Negative reinforcement, 90–91
Neuroticism, 37
Nurses: burnout in, 4, 7; conflict
among, 25; in palliative care set-
tings, 24; stress-reducing interventions for, 86–92; turnover
rate among, 10; turnover
replacement costs for, 9, 10

Nursing Stress Scale (NSS), 45–46

Occupations, most stressful, xii
Office of clinical effectiveness (OCE),
68
Oldenburg Burnout Inventory
(OLBI), 43, 48–49
"On the Folly of Rewarding A, While
Hoping for B" (Kerr), 82–83
Opportunities, for burnout reduc-
tion, identification of, 70, 71–72
Organizational culture: changes in,
28; for stress management, 75;
transmission through socializa-
tion programs, 88–89
Organizational factors, in burnout,
38–40, 41
Organizational performance, impact
of stress on, 8–12
Overeating, as response to stress, 6–7
Overtime: mandatory, 25
Overtime, mandatory, 56

Palliative care, 24
Participatory action research, 58
Partners, as coworkers, 83–84
Patient care, coordination of, 27–28
Patient outcomes, effect of physicians'
burnout on, 13
Patients, impact of healthcare staffs'
stress on, 12–14
Patient safety, 4
Patient satisfaction, decrease in, 14
Patients' demands, as stress cause,
24–25, 31
Perceived Stress Scale (PSS), 46
Performance appraisals: ineffective-
ness of, 90; negative behavior
focus of, 91; supportive behavior
component of, 83
Performance management, 90–91, 93
Personal factors, in burnout, 36,
37–39, 41
Personality traits, in burnout, 37, 41

Physical therapists, turnover replacement costs for, 9
Physician–patient relationship, lack of reciprocity in, 38–93
Physicians: conflict among, 25; stress experienced by, xiii; turnover replacement costs for, 9
Physiological measures, of stress, 44–45
Plan-Do-Check-Act quality improvement cycle, 59
Plan-Do-Study-Act quality improvement cycle, 59
Positive reinforcement, 90
PricewaterhouseCoopers' Health Research Institute, 10
Productivity: stress-related decrease in, 8, 11; turnover-related decrease in, 8–9
Professional development programs, 90

Quality improvement training, 29
Quality movement, in healthcare: as stress source, 26, 28–92; technology implementation in, 26

Realistic job previews (RJPs), 84, 86
Relationship building, in burnout reduction programs, 60, 61, 62–66, 68, 107
Resource(s): conservation of, 20–22, 31, 97; insufficient, xvi–xvii; motivational, 20–22, 31
Resource allocation: inadequate, 3; for medical error reporting, 13–14; secondary appraisal approach in, 19; strategic, 3
Resource investment, inadequate return on, 21–22, 31, 39
Resource management, 30–31
Respiratory therapists, turnover replacement costs for, 9
Rewards: for medical error reporting, 91; for supportive behavior,

82–83

Safety practices, negative effect of stress/burnout on, 4, 6, 7, 26
Schaufeli, Wilmar, 96
Scheduling: compressed workweeks, 92; flexible, 88; as source of stress, 25, 31
Self-organization, 98–99
September 11, 2001, 58
Shifts, overnight, 25, 62
Shirom, Arie, 6
Shirom-Melamed Burnout Measure, 49
Sincerity, of managers, 63, 64–65, 66
Sleep disturbances, burnout as risk factor for, 6
Smoking, 5–6
Social exchange model, of burnout, 38–93
Socialization programs, 88–89
Social Readjustment Scale, 44
Social support, work-related: emotional and instrumental, 81–82, 83, 99; meta-analysis of, 80–81; sources of, 37–38, 80–84
Sonographers, turnover rate among, 10
Spouses, as coworkers, 37–38, 83–84
Staff Burnout Scale for Health Professionals (SBS-HP), 50
Staffing, inadequate, 5, 25, 31
Staffing ratios, 86–88
Stakeholders, external, 67
Strain, 36, 61
Stress: adverse effects of, 5–6, xiii–xiv; as arousal, 1–2; assessment of, 31, 43–46, 51; causes of, xviii–xix; changes in attitudes toward, xiii; changes in reactions to, xiii; common consequences of, 2–7; contextual experience of, 44; definition of, xiv–xv; differentiated from dissatisfaction, xv–xvi; differenti-

ated from incompetence, xvi–xvii; differentiated from lack of commitment, xvi; economic impact of, 8–9; hypotheses regarding, 17–31; necessity of, 1–2; occupational, xii–xiv; organizational performance impact of, 8–12; patient care-related, 24–25; prevention of, 79–80; as subjective experience, xvii; transition to burnout, 35–40
"Stress balls," 56
Stress interviewing, 11
Stress management programs: failure of, xviii–xix; as individual interventions, xvii
Stressors: among administrative staff, 27–29; among clinical staff, 23–27, 31; appraisal of, 18–20, 31; avoidance of, 29–30, 41; as challenges, 69; commonality of, xviii; coping with, 19, 29–30, 41, xvii–xviii; definition of, xv; identification of, 62–63, 64–65, 66, 68–71; positive nature of, 44; pre-employment awareness of, 84–86; voluntary and involuntary, 44
Stress paradox, xvii–xix
Super-users, of technology, 72–73
Surgical departments, turnover-related costs in, 9
Surveys, 70
Sustainability: of burnout/stress reduction, 60, 61, 75–76, 79–93; expectations management for, 84–86; human resources management stress-reducing bundles for, 86–93; stress prevention for, 79–80

Teams, in burnout reduction programs, 66–68, 70–71, 75
Teamwork: crew resource management training in, 29; as organizational value, 83

Technology: as source of stress, 26–27, 31; super-user response to, 72–73
Tenure, 39–40
Time management programs, 54–55, 76
Training programs, 89–90
Transaction stress model, 18–20, 31
Turnover: burnout-related, 5, 6, 40; costs associated with, 8–11; non-stress-related reasons for, 10
Type A personality, 37

Unions, involvement in burnout reduction programs, 67
United Kingdom, most stressful jobs in, xii
University of Arizona, 9–10
University of Oklahoma, 86
University of Rhode Island, 86

Vacations, 76
Values, organizational, 88–89
Van Dierendonck, D. W. B., 57
Vigor, 96
Visibility, of managers, 63–64, 66

Wages, above-average, 91
Wheeler, Tony, 86–87
Work absences, 12
Workarounds, 3–4, 7; technology-related, 26, 27
Work environment, stress-free, 79–93; role of social support in, 80–84; role of stressor prevention in, 79–80
Workers' compensation, 12
Work–family conflict, 91–92
Work flow/processes, blocks in, 3–4, 27
Workload: control over, 38; as source of stress, 25, 31; structured for supportive behavior, 83
Workweek, compressed, 92

About the Author

Jonathon R. B. Halbesleben, PhD, is an assistant professor in the Department of Management and Marketing at the University of Wisconsin–Eau Claire, where he teaches undergraduate and graduate courses in healthcare management, organizational behavior, and human resources management.

Dr. Halbesleben has published more than 45 peer-reviewed articles based on his research on stress, burnout, engagement, and work–family relationships in such journals as the *Journal of Applied Psychology, Journal of Management, Medical Care, Medical Care Research and Review,* and *Health Care Management Review.* His research has garnered a number of awards, including Best Research-to-Practice Paper from the Health Care Management division of the Academy of Management in 2007. He is the editor of the *Handbook of Stress and Burnout in Health Care,* a scholarly compendium of current research on stress and burnout in the healthcare industry. He serves on the editorial boards of the *Journal of Organizational Behavior* and the *Journal of Management History* and is an associate editor of the *Journal of Occupational and Organizational Psychology.* He has received research funding from the Agency for Healthcare Research and Quality, the National Institute for Occupational Safety and Health, the U.S. Department of Defense, and the Centers for Disease Control and Prevention.

Dr. Halbesleben received his PhD and MS in industrial/organizational psychology from the University of Oklahoma and his BA in psychology from Winona State University. Prior to his position at the University of Wisconsin–Eau Claire, he worked in the School of Medicine at the University of Missouri and in the Michael F. Price College of Business at the University of Oklahoma.

Dr. Halbesleben is married to his lovely wife, Jennifer Becker, and has two children, Alex and Liesl. He is a native of Wisconsin and enjoys running, Brewers baseball, Packers and Sooners football, and playing with his kids.